Copyright © 2021 Jessica Portsmouth

All rights reserved

No part of this book may be reproduced, or stored in a retrieval system, or transmitted in any form or by any means, electronic, mechanical, photocopying, recording, or otherwise, without express written permission of the publisher.

This book does not replace the advice of a medical professional. Consult your physician before making any changes to your diet or regular health plan.

I have changed some names to protect individuals' privacy.

These are my memories, from my perspective, and I have tried to represent events as faithfully as possible.

The information in this book was correct at the time of publication, but the Author does not assume any liability for loss or damage caused by errors or omissions.

ISBN-13: 9780645338485

Cover design by: Bipolar Barbie

The Bipolar Barbie Diaries

✶✶✶

Volume 1

✶✶✶

DROWNING
in the Seas of Mental Illness

Bipolar Barbie

In loving memory of Joanne Murray, your love and support has never been forgotten. Your passing started this journey and as a result I continue it in your honour.

To my coaches and personal cheer squad

Aaron & Marrisa Armstrong

Zulu Flow Zion & the Flow Team

Crystal Frame & Amber Patterson

Sarah Nicole

Luana Ribeira

Emily & Ryan Berry

Grace McGurren

Alice Murray & TZ Perault

Jess Everson

Leah Sawell

Shaun Rotman

Tom Borg

Mum & Dad

Thank you for all of your guidance, support and believing in me even when I lost faith in myself.

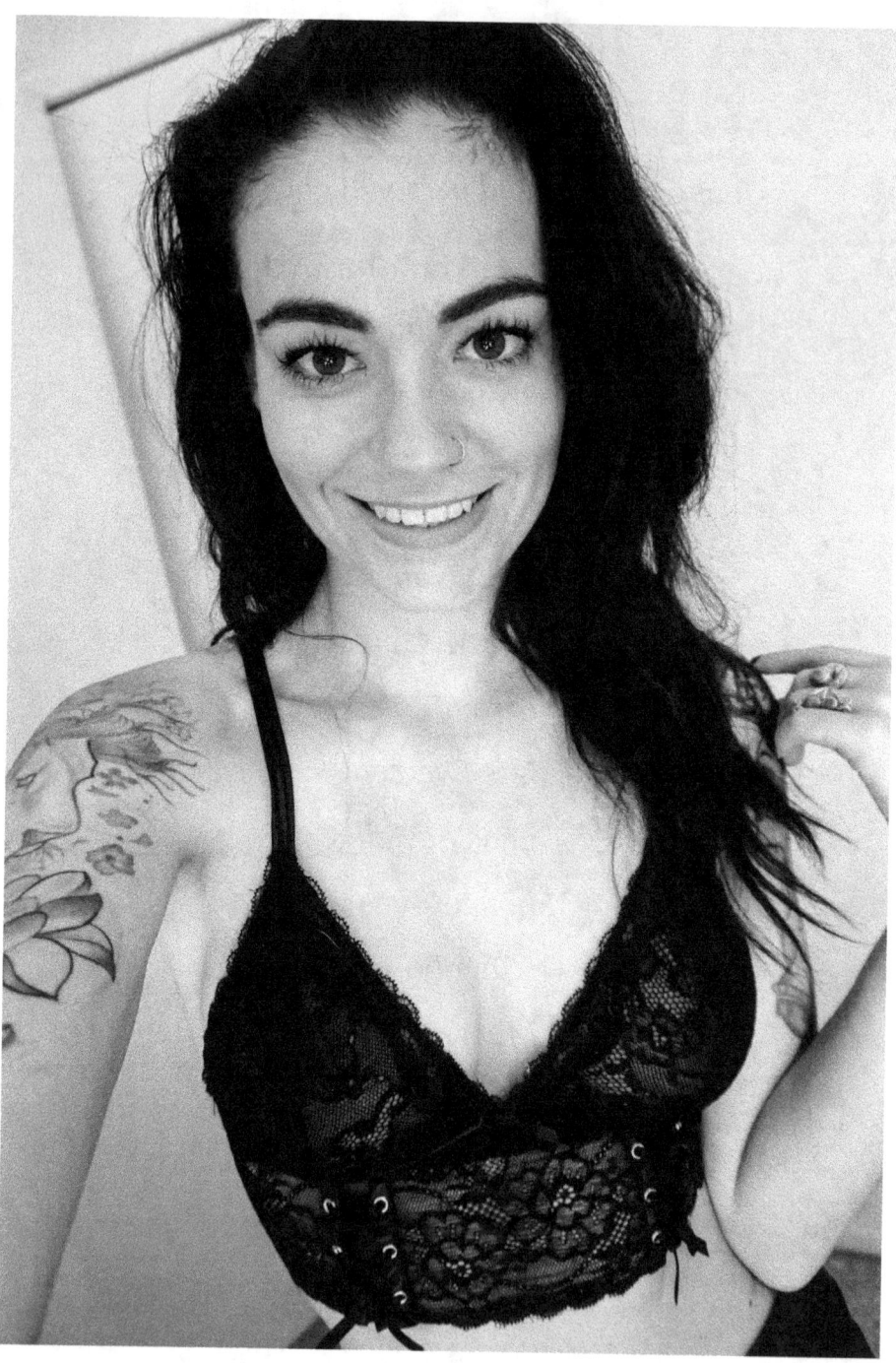

Why do I call myself Bipolar Barbie?

It all started during a severe manic episode in September of 2016, when my housemate asked me, "Why do you have so many clothes?"

I paused for a second, observing the war zone my room had become; I hadn't really noticed the mess up until she'd pointed it out. I guess I was too distracted by the flight of ideas swirling in my head and the exciting projects I had recently begun.

I had no idea the 'floordrobe' in my cave had expanded to such impressive heights. With shock, and a subtle hint of pride, I realised my floor resembled more of a Himalayan mountain ridge than a bedroom. The sea of clothes spilling over from one pile to another, merging both clean and dirty, formed such a mass it could rival the island of trash accumulating in the middle of the Pacific Ocean.

The thought of cleaning up this natural disaster sent shivers down my spine. This clothes spill seemed to be more daunting than the very real possibility that I was losing my mind. I wondered to myself how this could have happened. I had a flashback to digging through my closet, trying to find something to wear that was even remotely agreeable. Nothing felt right at the time. It was as if the clothes weren't mine – as if I was raiding someone else's wardrobe.

Then it hit me. I have so many different clothes because I have so many different personalities, each in need of their own wardrobe! My outfits are an external expression of how I feel. It's an extension of the mood state I am in. It's almost like I could use each day's outfit as a mood ring, sometimes changing dramatically from Tuesday to Wednesday.

But with each, I was reminded of the Barbie doll I'd had when I was a kid and how extensive her wardrobe was. I suddenly empathized with her for not being able to pick her own outfits. I not only decided what she wore, but who she would be each day. I felt sorry for Barbie. I related to her in an entirely different way. She had her default personas like Dr. Barbie, Roller Skating Barbie, Ballerina Barbie, Malibu Barbie, and a huge variety of other occupations and hobbies.

The more I thought about it, the more I realised I was a lot like her; but my personas were Manic Barbie, Suicidal Barbie, Anxious Barbie, Depressed Barbie, Borderline Barbie, Self-Harming Barbie, Fatigued Barbie, PMDD Barbie, Migraine Barbie and any other combination of symptoms my mental illnesses decided to make me deal with each day. I was literally a Bipolar Barbie doll. I had my outfits, and, like Barbie, I was being dressed by some other force I didn't quite understand. I was at the will of my illness and it dressed me each day however it saw fit, forcing me to play a role along with it.

Sometimes I would rapidly change throughout the day and due to the limitations of my financial circumstances and wardrobe, I always seemed to be living a life I was never dressed appropriately for. I was roller Skating Barbie at the banquet, Ballerina Barbie in the courtroom, Horse Riding Barbie getting married, Scuba Diving Barbie in the desert, and Sleeping Barbie under water. It never felt right. I was always a different version of myself. I couldn't help but wonder, who was Naked Barbie anyway?

Unfortunately, unlike Barbie, I didn't get a new life each game. I didn't get a break when the girl dropped her toys. There was no mother to pick up the scattered dolls off the floor, packing them and their accessories into a crowded container before stuffing it under the bed. Although I could relate to the suffocating feeling of being trapped in a box full of anticipation and dread, half dressed, surrounded by the debris of my possessions waiting for play time to end and the five year old demons to go to bed.

I couldn't hit reset whenever I wanted. I had all these different personas and had to live the same life; a life meant for one person in each body. I had multiple people living within me and each of them had their own versions. I was constantly swapping and changing, it's no wonder I found it hard to maintain any form of stability.

I choose to view my mental illnesses as filters that are applied to my life. As entities outside of myself that get wrapped around me like cloaks so that I can one day learn how to take them off.

The truth is, I don't expect this book to make much sense. The truth is, I am telling a story I don't yet quite understand.

Mental illness is a general term for a range of conditions which affect a person's mood, behaviour or thinking. With a current diagnosis of Bipolar Disorder type 2, Borderline Personality Disorder and Premenstrual Dysphoric Disorder, how can anything I do be rational or make perfect sense yet?

There are moments in my life where things move left, right, backwards, diagonally, and don't quite connect. My mind fast forwards and rewinds at the same time. I try to be consistent but that is hard when you are stuck in a washing machine on a heavy duty spin cycle.

They say life is a journey not a race and I think recovery is a way of life not a place. Mental illness has no itinerary and this expedition does not either. Trust me, we both have questions, and things will escalate quickly.

I will admit, at times I lose touch with reality. Sometimes I get so caught up in my head, the fabrications of my messed up mind seem real to me. *What is 'real' anyway? The perception of events widely accepted by most? Am I the only one that feels this way? Is it true what they say? Am I crazy?*

It may seem trivial to you. But this is my truth. My reality and my twisted and tangled story. It is a complex web that weaves its way back and forth. It's a maze even the brightest of minds like Einstein and Da Vinci likely could not fathom to understand. It's like my life was shattered one day. All I have done since is try to put the incomplete puzzle pieces back together.

It may not be a complete picture. But it is the most accurate picture of me at the time of writing this. It may seem jumbled or at times incomplete, but I have hope that someone who is seeking help with their mental illness might be able to pick up a volume and read a few entries to feel less alone in this world.

These books are simply a compilation of my own personal diaries. They give a glimpse into the thought processes and inner dialogue in my mind. They express my own thoughts and feelings about my life.

Names, places and details may have been changed to protect the privacy of others. Anything written within these pages is nothing more than my own personal opinion. I am not a doctor or a trained mental health professional. My only qualifications are 'lived experience'. Any reference to medical conditions, medication or anything else is only written in context of my own personal understanding and experiences on the subject matter.

This journal could be read in many ways. It isn't a finished story but a journey of self-discovery, and that never really ends does it?

Please don't judge my story by the chapter you walked in on. I have volumes of this stuff. This is just part 1. So, if you're as confused as a chameleon in a bag of skittles, then we are on the same page!

Bipolar Barbie

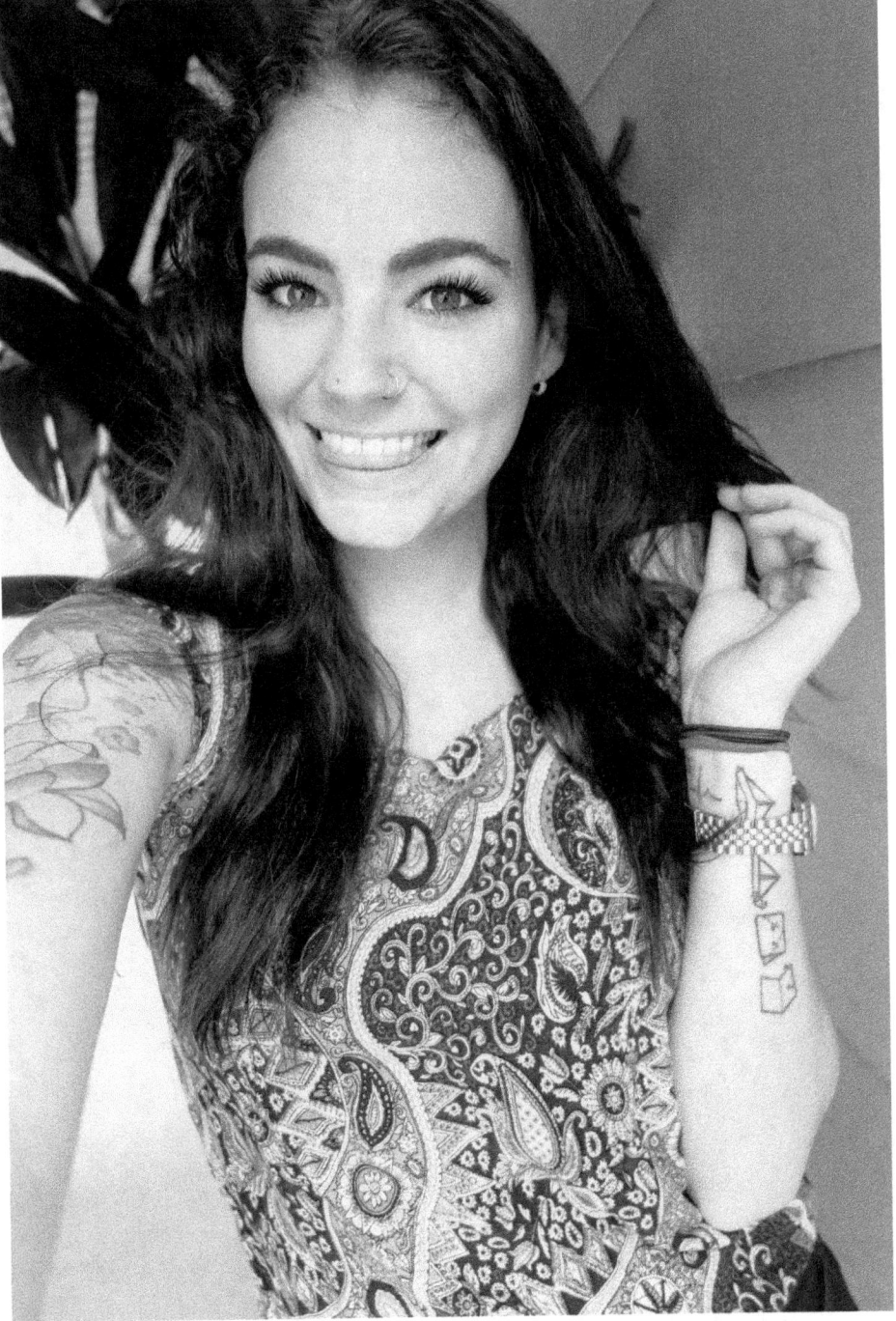

Grief comes and goes in waves. If I stop now, I might just drown in the sea of my own grief.

Bipolar Barbie

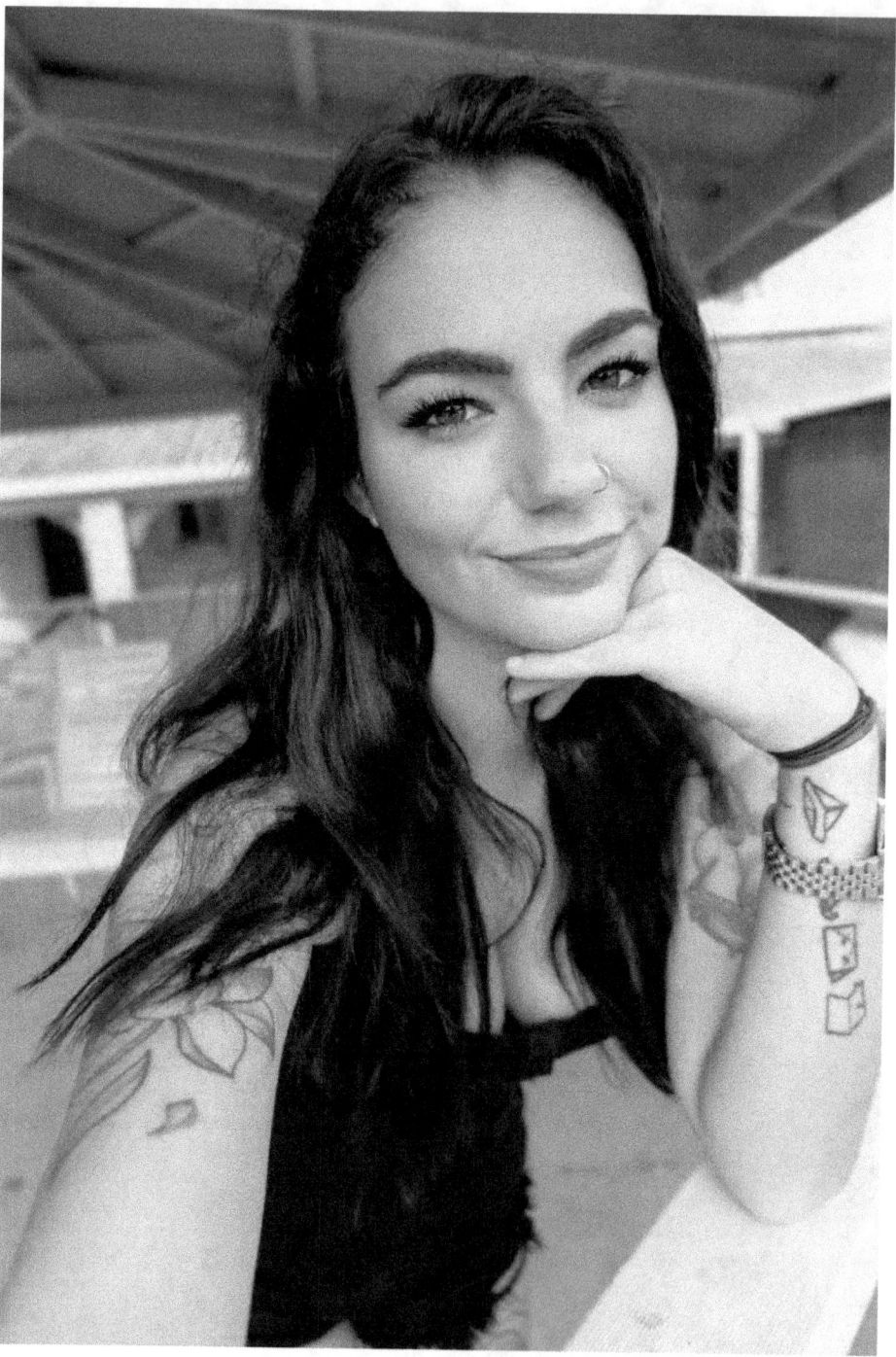

Dear Diary,

I still remember the day my entire life changed. I was in my second year of Law School, about to collapse on the floor of my dorm room, when I realized my life would never be the same again. At the time, I didn't know exactly what changed, but I felt like I was Dorothy in *The Wizard Of Oz*. I had no idea where I was, I just knew that I wasn't in Kansas anymore.

It was like that movie Freaky Friday, starring Lindsay Lohan and Jamie Lee Curtis, where they switched bodies overnight. I seemed to not be in my own body anymore. I was possessed. I was screaming at myself, trying to get control of the wheel, but I was unsuccessful. I was a fly on the wall of my dorm room trying to get the attention of this unknown occupant. I was floating above myself not recognising the creature inside my physical form.

I couldn't shake the feeling of a foreboding presence standing over me. I felt I was imploding. I was too heavy, and I was fading away; being dragged into this black hole that appeared in the pit of my stomach. I felt like I was eating myself from the inside out. I was being devoured by this evil force within. It was like my soul was haemorrhaging into this foreign abyss.

The worst part was, I felt alone in all this. No one else could hear the things the walls whispered to me or the way the night screamed my name. The moon beckoned me to come home, as it glowed in the night sky like a beacon showing me the way. I howled like a wolf knowing a strange change was in the air.

I wondered if I had fallen through the time space continuum and landed in an alternate reality? I felt like the Flash, accidentally running too fast and bursting through the multiverse to another earth. Everything looked the same, but nothing felt right. *How did I get here? I wondered. Where am I? Can I really be in another plane of existence? Am I dreaming? Is this a nightmare? It has to be! No one's reality can be this bleak.*

The last thing I remember was being in Perth visiting my childhood friend George for Spring break. I remember feeling on top of the world. She introduced me to CrossFit and Olympic weightlifting. I trained at her gym, while she taught classes, and the rest of the time we spent at the beach talking and laughing for hours on end. It reminded me of a much simpler time. We were fourteen again, sitting on the hill at lunch watching the clouds roll in. I didn't want to go home. She offered me the chance to stay and live with her and her fiancé, but I declined because I wanted to finish my law degree.

I loved law. It was my dream job. I was born to take on a court room and make the law my bitch. I could argue before I could walk and talk shit with marbles in my mouth underwater according to my mother. I loved memorising legal statutes, negotiating settlements and most of all, defending a client in front of a judge. In only two short years I would be a fully qualified practising Criminal Defence attorney. By twenty-five I would have bought my own home and be earning $100,000 a year. By thirty I would be a senior partner in a prestigious law firm and married to the man of my dreams with two kids. By thirty-five I would become a judge. My life was on track … if everything went according to plan that is. But nothing ever does, does it?

In September 2012 I had never been so clear headed, motivated, and focused. I was ready to return to Uni with this inspired gust of wind beneath my wings. I was a bird ready to take flight, and I was sure I was about to reach new heights.

But a phone call cut my trip short and marked the beginning of the end for me. My father asked me to hop on the next plane home because my grandmother had just passed away. I agreed to get on the next flight, and meet my uncle in Sydney, who would drive me to the funeral. The next couple of days were a blur of black outfits, sombre faces, and murmured condolences. It was a shock compared to the upbeat pace my delightful Spring break had set.

I was excited to return to University and be reunited with my fun, new, excited tone. No one at University would remind me of those last couple of days of my holidays. I could start fresh. A new me, a new semester, and new opportunities awaited me, just a four-hour drive from my parent's house. I let the drive wash away the end of my holiday and re-energize me as I headed towards the Sunshine Coast.

I arrived back in the dorms and was greeted with friendly faces. Campus was abuzz with students returning, and it seemed like we all were eager to get back to our routines. I felt a sigh of relief the moment I opened the door to my dorm room and was greeted by my artwork-adorned walls. *Home sweet home,* I thought. With barely a moment to rest, I put my bags down and started receiving guests at my door. Finally, things were back to normal. The sunshine and sweet, fresh Gold Coast air was like satin, skimming over my olive skin. The golden sandstone buildings of Bond University had never looked more appealing. Life was perfect. I had everything I ever dreamt of – great friends, a scholarship to law school, a beautiful place to live, and a job to pay for my accommodation. I was happy, healthy, and fitter than ever.

After catching up on each other's holidays, I got straight into my new routine. Gym, study, socializing. I had it all planned out on a time blocked schedule colour coded and everything. I was determined to make this semester my best yet. I was going to get out more and meet new people. Join the rowing club and make the most of my university experience. I was stoked on my high grades from last semester and I wanted to do even better. But the universe had something else planned for me.

No one could have predicted the turn my first week back at Uni would take. A friend of mine was found dead in her bed the morning after our first 'Welcome Back' pub crawl. My heart sank to the pit of my stomach as the news quickly spread through the campus grapevine. It felt like sour wine fermenting in our mouths. We were all affected by the loss of one of our friends. But it was like our grief shared made it easier to digest. The dispersal of our loss made it less intense for each of us to bear.

I had lost close friends before; growing up in the town that had the highest youth suicide rate and car accident fatality count in all of Australia, meant you became well-acquainted with terrible, tragic losses. As frequent as they were, I don't think you ever got used to them. In fact, I think they hurt more each time, like a compounding grief you could in no way shake. You never forget the mornings you are called into the principal's office or ushered with the rest of your classmates to the school hall, to be told that a friend, at fourteen, had seen no other alternative to escape the abuse of his step-father, than to kill himself. Or that a girl you used to play Bratz dolls with and celebrated birthdays with, since you were just tiny pre-schoolers, had been decapitated in a truck accident. Or being driven home from dancing in a torrential rainstorm, to see a mass of police and emergency workers desperately searching for your neighbour, who you waited at the bus stop with each day for school for the past five years. To pray for days that he is found alive – cold and shaken, but alive – and seeing them pack up three days later, after finding his body trapped under a submerged log. Or to hear that your piano teacher had jumped off a quarry. That a friend you used to horse ride with was killed on his motorbike, or the girl you used to compete on the debating team with, and mess around at recess with, had died under mysterious circumstances. But despite my previous losses, and the two in the past week – the next one would be the third in a month – this one was going to change my life forever.

    I remember pre-drinking in my common room for our official 'Welcome Back' University party. It was the first night that everyone had returned, and classes were due to start on Monday. 'Shot Roulette' was followed by 'Goon of Fortune' and 'King's Cup'. We blared throwback tunes from our portable speakers. We danced on the couches and poured drinks all over the tables. "Teenage Dirtbag" by Wheatus had just come on as I checked my phone to call us a taxi, stopping to read a text message from Ally, my best friend's older sister. She told me that her mum had just suffered a stroke. One of the boys at the party asked me if I was okay, and I told him what had happened. He said he was sober and offered to drive me home immediately. I told him the four-hour drive wasn't necessary; I'd talked with Ally, and I'm not sure if it was my drunk state or her understatement of the situation, but I'd had the impression it wasn't serious. How wrong I was.

I partied until the early hours of the morning, completely forgetting the conversation. It wasn't until I was awoken by the splitting headache late in the morning, that I thought I should call to check in. But before I pulled myself together, the phone rang. It was Mr. Mac. He had never called me before, though I knew him well after living with him and their family for years.

Mamma JoJo always referred to me as her fifth daughter. Her house was a safe haven for orphans and rejects like me. She took me in when my own parents didn't want me. She nurtured me and mothered me in a way I had never experienced. She was a mother goose to so many wayward souls. She had a way of making the broken feel whole again and helping the lost feel at home.

When the strong biker club president spoke, I noticed he wasn't his normal strong self. He was distraught. I could hear the tears in his eyes. He told me that Mum had a stroke and was in a medically-induced coma. She had fallen whilst making a cup of tea in the kitchen and had not been conscious since. He said it was bad and urged me to come home to say my goodbyes. In shock, I stood frozen with the phone in my hand. I couldn't move. I was solid like a rock, but I knew the moment I flinched, I'd collapse under the weight of this disturbing news. I opened my dorm room door and was greeted by my dorm mates in the hallway. They were laughing and reminiscing over last night's shenanigans – a conversation I would usually have happily joined – until one of them noticed something was wrong. I couldn't speak the words. They wouldn't come out. I fell to the floor, and Ana caught me as I sunk into the carpet. I started wailing hysterically. No one knew what was going on. I knew the moment I shared what had happened it would be real. I didn't want it to be. Through heavy sobs, I managed to utter the truth. Shocked faces greeted my admission and arms fell around me. I was glad they were there to hold me together … but it wouldn't last long.

I fell apart that day. I shattered into a thousand shards I was sure were too sharp to put back together. I was broken beyond repair. Something snapped, like a glow stick being cracked. The lights came on, but then rapidly flickered on and off. Total darkness one second would suddenly become illuminated, with the brightest of magical, white light. Before long, it was an all-night long strobe party in my brain. Fireworks and all. Maybe it was the straw that broke the camel's back or perhaps this was part of the master plan all along. All I know is that from that day on, I was no more.

I died the moment I watched the life drain out of the eyes of my surrogate mother. I held her hand while she took her last breaths. It was surreal. I felt like I was in a Salvador Dali painting as time slipped away. Clocks were melting as the days turned into weeks, and I turned to alcohol to numb the pain. I lost my life-support the moment they switched off hers. I was forced to add another anniversary to a calendar full of dates I'd rather forget.

I used the distance from home and the secluded world of my University campus to distract myself from real life. I spent less time at home and lived a lie, convincing myself I was fine. A white lie that I told so many times, I perhaps started to believe it. I didn't feel like I had a right to be so sad. She wasn't my real mother, although she felt like the most real one I'd had. I distracted my mind, keeping myself busy with a huge class load, extracurricular activities, and social gatherings. I became a social butterfly. Soon, everyone knew my name. I was praised for being so sociable ... but they didn't know that I had to distract myself from what was going on inside. I needed to be distracted. I was terrified of being alone. The pain was unbearable.

I tried harder than ever to be happy. When I was dancing on a table at a club or slurping spilled vodka off a bar, the crowd would cheer, and the sound of their applause would take me to a better place. But as the attention died down, I would come crashing back to reality. I'd look around and see the smiles of everyone else in the room, having a good time and I would once again be heavy and hollow in my deep-rooted sorrow. I just wanted to feel whole again. When I was by myself, I feared being alone with my thoughts. Never before had I been so distraught.

After a while, my tears ran dry. I couldn't cry anymore. Who knew you could feel such great pain and so numb all at the same time? I was dry and brittle like a statue carved out of pumice stone. I tried to hydrate myself. I spent weeks curled up on the floor of the communal dorm showers until the water ran cold, often covered in my own vomit from the alcohol I'd hide in my room and consume when I needed to escape. Which was always. I hid my daily habit under the illusion of a Uni student just having a good time. Everyone believed it, because no one knew the depths of my dirty little secret; I always had a bottle of tequila on my bedside table. I'd keep a sour lemon and salt shaker on hand, just so I could start drinking before I even got out of bed.

I was going through the motions of my daily routine on autopilot. I felt like a puppet with broken strings. No matter how hard I pulled, my body just lay lifeless at my feet. I didn't know what to feel. I just stared at the ceiling, like I was floating on a cloud. I felt like I had been injected with numbing agents like at the dentist. Somehow, it had infiltrated my entire body. My tongue and cheeks wouldn't listen to me when I told them to smile. My eyes wouldn't close when I asked them to sleep. I was absent. I was a stranger to myself. Everyone acted like I was the same person, but I wasn't *her* anymore. I was none of the things I used to be. I had lost everything that made me *me*.

The high school student with impeccable grades, multi-discipline sporting champion, debating captain, national public speaker, and Miss Universe contestant seemed like a figment of my imagination. Had I been deluded all these years? Were all those award ceremonies, trophies, and newspaper feature articles on me fake? Were they a dream or was this a nightmare? How else could I explain that the person who was good at everything, who could achieve anything she set her mind to, could barely get out of bed? Was the promise of being 'most likely to succeed' a lie?

Nothing had ever been hard for me in my life. Even as a sixteen-year-old, embarking on a twelve-month student exchange program to a foreign country was a walk in the park compared to this. I had never found a riddle that I couldn't work out. This was a problem that needed solving and fast! But what on earth was wrong? I was lost, that was clear. But where was I exactly? There was no map, there was no city. Nothing but a maze in a twisted world that didn't seem so normal anymore. I was Alice watching myself disappear down a rabbit hole into a not so wonderful place.

It all happened so suddenly. One day, I knew exactly who I was and the next day that girl was gone.

POOF!

She had vanished. Just like water droplets evaporating into thin air, she was gone without a trace. I tried to track her down, but it was like chasing a phantom. A whisper of a legend that perhaps once lived. I turned over every stone in search of who I once was, but it was like she never even existed. The only reason I knew she was real, was because everyone else still compared me to her. The worst part was that no one really believed she was gone.

At first, I mourned my past self, but soon I began to hate her. How could she leave me? Why did she abandon me? I hated her for the obnoxious, over-achieving, insanely perfect, talented, smart, beautiful and popular girl she was. I was jealous of her. I suddenly realised how most people probably viewed me at school. Did they all love to secretly hate me? Did I fill them with the same envious resentment I felt towards her now?

They all seemed to know her well, a little too well. Perhaps better than I did. The picture they painted was of a wonderful person, who I am sure anyone would dream of being. I never thought she was perfect at the time, but compared to this mess, she seemed like a goddess, walking divinely on this Earth. Why would I willingly throw her away?

Before I had time to adjust to this new me, I had to convince everyone else I was different. It was like trying to convince a bunch of sceptics that I was a time traveller or a person from another dimension. I was merely a doppelgänger or stunt double for my once vibrant self. I was the understudy of an actress playing the lead suddenly thrust into the spotlight without learning my lines. I was centre stage with the bright spotlight on, in shock. The crowd all stared at me expectantly with anticipation and adoration that quickly turned into impatience and disdain. I was playing a beloved character with no idea how to act. Every step or action I took was wrong. I had no idea what was going on.

I felt like a parent trying to convince the police my child had been kidnapped, but instead of investigating that lead, they just accused me of being the murderer, and refused to see it any other way. I think I would have had more luck convincing someone that a dingo ate my baby, than I did trying to tell them the old me was missing. They just looked at me with confused expressions and tried to convince me that because my physical body was right in front of them, it meant my mind was too. Everyone seemed to look at me in disbelief, like I had lost my mind!

The truth was, I had.

No one prepares you for what it will be like if you are the one in four unlucky enough to lose your mind. No one teaches you what to do or who to turn to if, and when it happens. To be honest ... I don't think anyone really knows. No one tells you that once you have lost your mind, you might continue losing it time and time again. No matter how many times you think you have found it. It slips through your fingers easier than you think. It's pretty apparent when you have lost it, but not always clear when you have regained it. What does it mean to be sane anyway?

I have spent the last ten years chasing my sanity and yet I still haven't figured out how you can lose something so internal, something that is a part of yourself and plays a vital role in our basic human survival. I always ask myself *why?* How can our brains be so evolved but yet so weak, vulnerable and at times broken or be just plain defective? Do animals go insane? If it is true that I have lost my mind, where has it gone? Did I ever have it in the first place? How did the few screws loose in my head come undone? Or were they always rattling around? I don't know. But I do remember the day I heard them for the first time. None of that seems to matter now. All I care about is putting them back in their place so I can function like the well-oiled machine I once was.

Now I'm searching for some magical reality called recovery. I hear that's where I will be reunited with my sanity. Does it even really exist though? What is a 'sane' person, and do I even want to be one? If my sanity is hidden, then contrary to popular belief, it *was* locked away. Out of sight, out of my mind … I knew I had to get it back, but I lacked the resources to enlist help in finding it. I also didn't know what resources were available … no one did.

It has been a long and treacherous journey so far. One that I am still embarking on. The worst part is no one believes it's real. So no one helps me. I feel like Dora the Explorer asking for advice through a TV screen. Maybe I would have a better chance at convincing children my demons exist. Most people don't believe I need help because they supposedly can't see it ...

No one understands what I am talking about when I ask for help. It's like I am trying to convince them that I am the Messiah or have supernatural powers like X-ray vision. If I am being honest though, I never thought this would ever happen to me until it did. So it doesn't surprise me that no one else believed it could have happened to me either.

Perhaps the hardest part in convincing others of how very real my predicament is, is because I don't know exactly what I have lost. I try desperately to search every part of this earth for what I think I lost. I reject things that no longer make me happy (which seems to be everything) and search for new opportunities that might evoke a sense of happiness inside me. But to no avail. It is true what they say that you don't realise what you have until it's gone. You don't know the value of your sanity until one day you wake up and it's nowhere to be found. Just like that you're someone else. a different person. And I didn't like who she was.

I have since come to the conclusion that *I* am the problem. It isn't my life that is broken, it is me. I am defective. A sad realization I have had to finally accept; that I am the root of all evil. My Dad must be secretly rejoicing, "I told you so, young demon child!"

Although broken, I have begun to reflect on my life as I try to hold on to what little I have left. The first I am rather good at, the later not so much ... I am grasping at bubbles in water trying to catch what little parts of me that remain as they slowly drift beyond my reach. Regrettably I have thrown things away I never wanted to lose. I have jumped to conclusions that should have never been made. Although I often blame myself ... I haven't been in control of myself for a long time either. I don't know what or who is ... but it's certainly not me.

I watch myself and my life fall apart from a high vantage point, like a gargoyle perched precariously atop a haunted house. I have a stunning bird's-eye view of the world's worst horror film imaginable. A horror film that just so happens to be my life. I am scared. I desperately keep trying to battle my demons and fight my way through the war in my head, hoping the enemy has the key to finding what I have lost. After all, weren't they the ones that took it away?

I don't know how long I expected this war to last ... but it was definitely meant to be over by now. At this point, I fear that no matter how much fight I have within me ... the enemy may outlast me. I live in fear of that moment when all hope is lost for good, and I cannot muster the courage to summon every bit of strength I have. Yet somehow, although defeated every day ... I am still alive. I am yet to decide whether or not that is a good thing. Am I being punished? Or tested? Does it matter?

I am adrift in the rough seas of mental illness and have been for years. I am at the mercy of the changing tide and strong, moody currents. I am tormented by storms that always seem to be brewing on the horizon. When the hurricanes of mania and torrential rain of depression hit, I wonder what hope there is for me? How can I signal help? Who can help me? Why is this happening to me? What did I do to deserve this? I don't want to die, but I don't see any other way out. I'm terrified of drowning, but it seems inevitable now. The very real possibility of drowning out here alone sinks in and I don't know how much longer I can keep myself afloat. Each day, I become a little more exhausted, disorientated, petrified, and adrift in the vast unknown. I have no idea what lurks in the water below. It's dark and cold. I'm not sure what I am more afraid of; is it what could be circling below ... or being out here alone?

All I know is that I was in a world I didn't understand, like Dorothy in *The Wizard of Oz*. All I wanted was to go home. But with nothing on the horizon in every direction, I felt more like Toto running into the witch's den. I had no idea what the hell was going on, let alone how to fix it. But I had to. I couldn't live like this anymore. That I knew for sure. I could not take one more minute of this hell. I desperately needed to rid myself of whatever had possessed my body. I had to get back to shore, but I had no idea where the shore was. I needed to find my destination before I could head towards it. I had to know the problem before I could fix it. I had to know where to begin. But no one I knew could tell me any more than I already knew.

In the beginning, I watched everybody around me go about their business, floating safely in boats. It was like I was encased in a soundproof glass box. I was there, but nobody really noticed. I must have been invisible. I had to be. Why else would they ignore my cries for help? I was drowning, and I needed help. I was gasping for air, suffocating. I couldn't breathe. I was growing more exhausted by the minute. I was standing right in front of them, clearly in trouble, but no one seemed to notice … how could they not? I tried as hard as I could to get their attention. I reached out. I swam toward them and tried my best to get them to notice me.

"I'm drowning!" I screamed, "I need your help!" But I was only ever met with blank expressions that quickly turned away. No one wanted to help me. I had no idea why, but it made me feel even worse. I managed to keep my head above water, but my heart sank. Why did they let me go? The ones I loved could see my struggle – I knew they could.

The only logical explanation was that no one believed I was worth saving. I would dive into the coldest, deepest, darkest of waters to rescue the ones I love, but no one offered the same courtesy to me. I thought it meant they didn't love me, that I wasn't worth anything to them. It gave me the impression that my life wasn't worth saving in their eyes. It broke me.

But, I persisted, and continued to try my best to convince those around me that I needed help. What else are loved ones for?

Insane Barbie

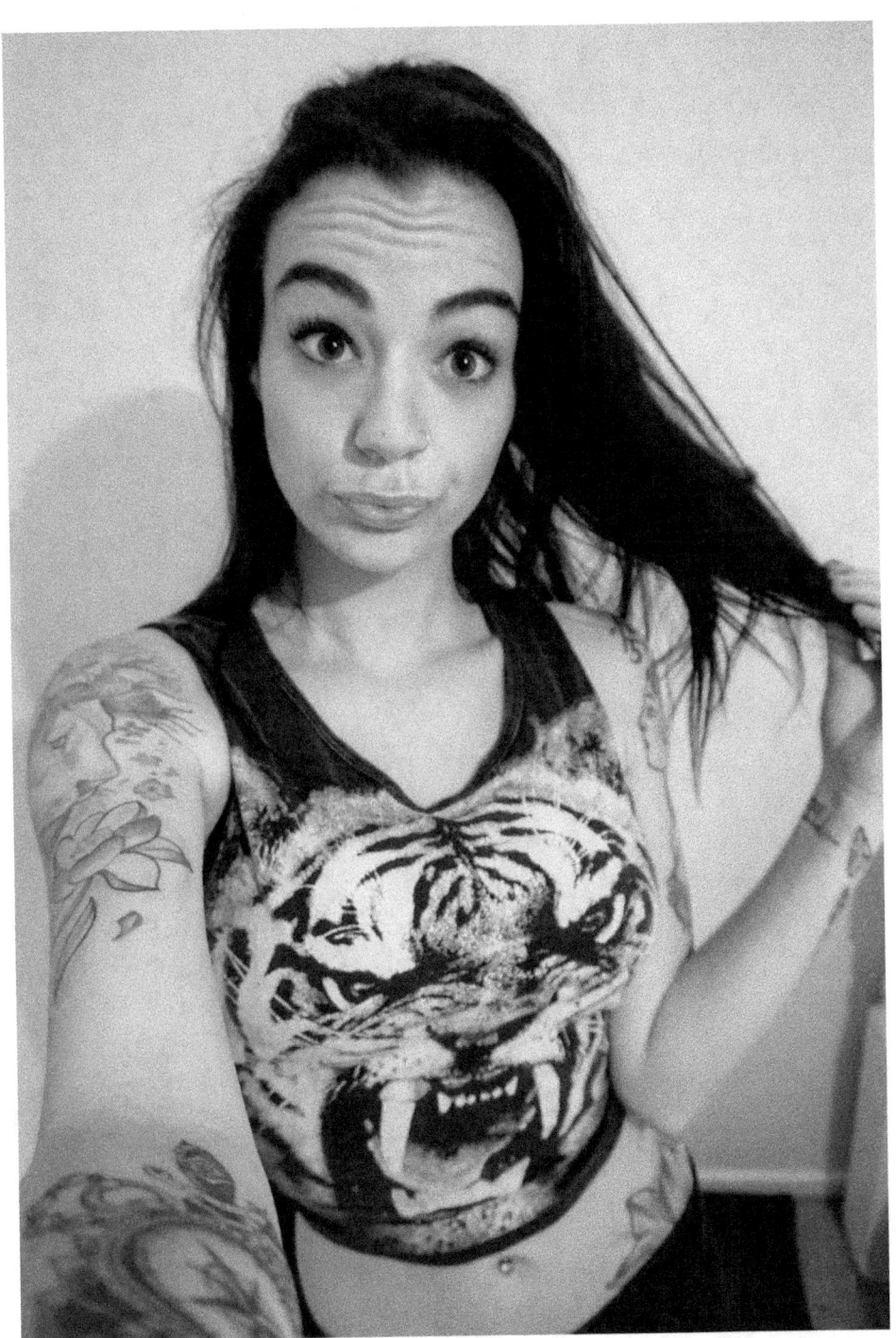

*The whirlpool of emotions sucked me dry
until the ocean of grief became a glittering
night sky.*

Bipolar Barbie

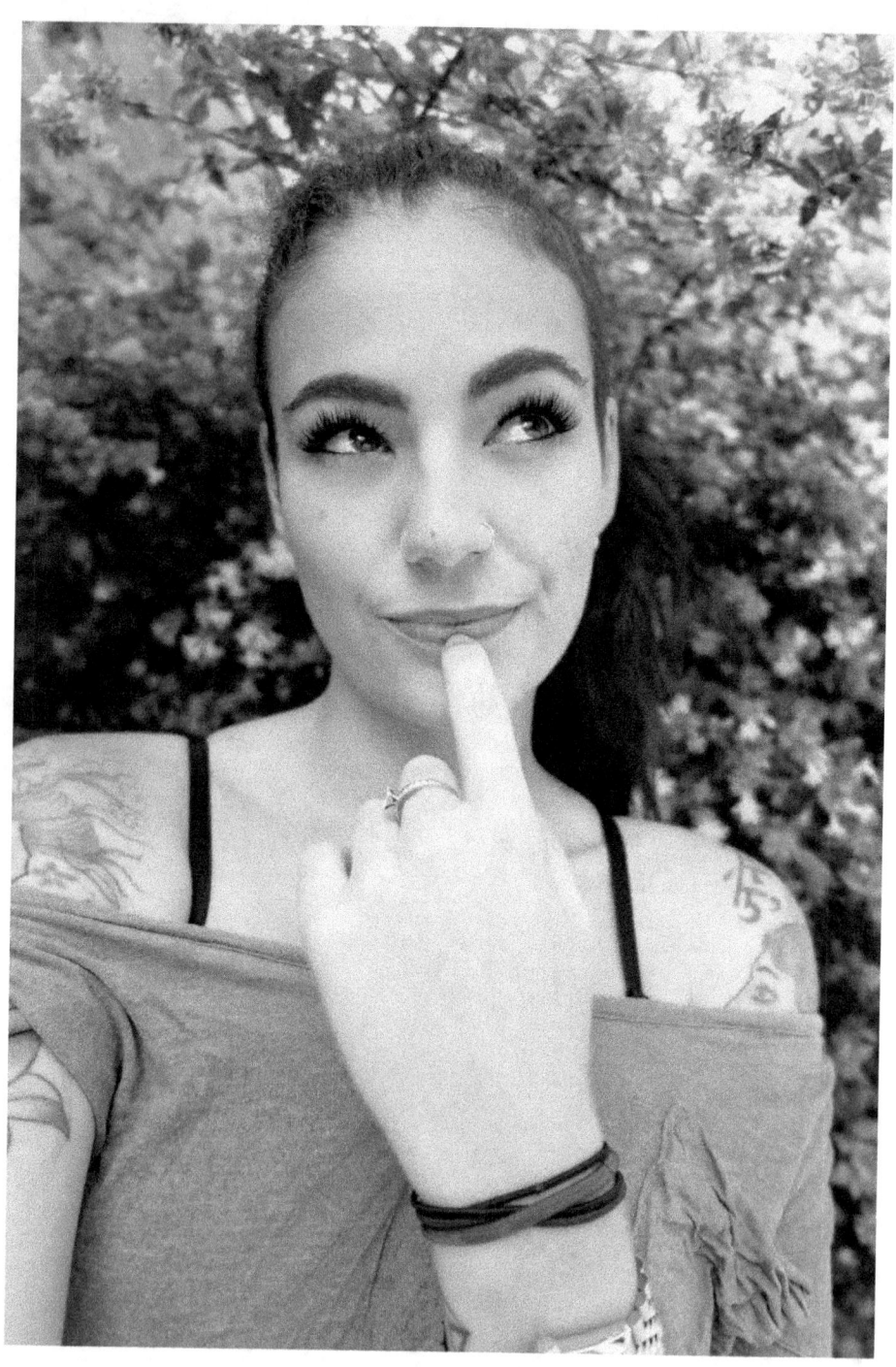

Dear Diary,

Have I lost my mind?

How does one lose their mind? Is it a twisted fate that brings such misery to a person? Or are they victims of their own mistakes? Why have I been chosen to bear this curse? What have I done to deserve such a harsh punishment?

I am desperately searching everywhere I can think of for answers, but time is running out. My health is deteriorating more rapidly each day, and it seems to be a race against the clock. Will I find a cure for whatever ailment has befallen me before it takes me away forever? Will it kill me, or will it just bring me to the brink of death and hold me over the edge for the rest of my days?

I am in a state of disbelief while I desperately search for relief. I feel like I have been pushed out of a helicopter and dropped into the middle of the ocean, in the dead of the night. I don't remember how I got here; it is like someone kidnapped me in my sleep, knocked me out, tied me up, blindfolded me, flew as far out into the Pacific Ocean as they could, and threw me out of the aircraft, leaving me there to die. I am terrified, cold, and worst of all, alone. My world has suddenly frozen over like Arendelle in an endless winter. I am Elsa, escaping my own wrath. Everything I touch withers up and dies. I am trapped in a snow globe, bobbing about in the sea like a message in a bottle. The only trouble is the glass is some sort of filtered mirror. People only see what they want to see; a beautiful girl, wasting her 'potential'. From their perspective, the glass is so transparent that it doesn't even exist. They don't notice the message I am shouting from the rooftops, "I am not okay!".

I think day and night about lighting a fire the size of an inferno you could see from space, hoping someone will see it and rescue me. Like a fire lit by a marooned sailor on an island trying to grab the attention of a passing ship. It doesn't work. "Why?" I desperately ask.

Maybe I can't manifest the flint and kindling or maybe I just think I am so visible that it isn't necessary to create such a ruckus or fuss? I have tested the waters a couple of times, I've sent smoke signals, and hoped they'd realise that where there's smoke, there's usually fire. But everyone just grows tired of the smell of smoke. I get asked politely to stop fanning it in their direction. People shy away from me as if protecting themselves from poisonous fumes. I feel toxic as I walk around in a haze of smog.

Apparently, there's a time limit on grief. As the months go by, sincere condolences about the loss of Jo soon turn into reassurances that I will feel better soon, and then to polite encouragement to move on.

Eventually they issue final demands to build a bridge and to just get over it before leaving me for dead.

"We all have issues, people die," they tell me. They act like I am deliberately prolonging the grieving process of the most important person in my life because I enjoy being distraught. The truth is, I don't know how not to be anymore.

When I confide in those around me that Jo wasn't my biological mother, it seems their empathy towards her passing is drastically reduced. Blood was never what defined my family, but it is clear that others don't see it that way. Some people cannot comprehend the reasons someone might be abandoned by their own tribe. Maybe I can blame their privilege on that. I am attending Australia's most expensive university after all. The only reason I am here is because I won a scholarship. It's no surprise I can barely relate to a bunch of trust fund babies who get an allowance worth more than my car every week. How could they possibly understand what it was like to be cared for by a surrogate mother when your own couldn't stand you?

We all grieve differently, and we all have different upbringings. When people evaluate the relative impact death has on us, titles we give the people in our lives seem to rank them higher than the role they played. The trust fund babies at the University can't comprehend someone on a scholarship, working simultaneously to pay their own way through Law School. They couldn't understand the concept of a broken home and fractured parental-child relationships. But they could comprehend the loss of a birth mother. As if pushing someone out of your vagina makes you a Mother. Motherhood is a title, being a mother is a choice. Some throw the right to that title out the moment they give birth.

    I don't know how long it takes a person to "get over" such a tragic loss. I haven't seemed to get over it. I don't know if I ever will.

Grieving Barbie

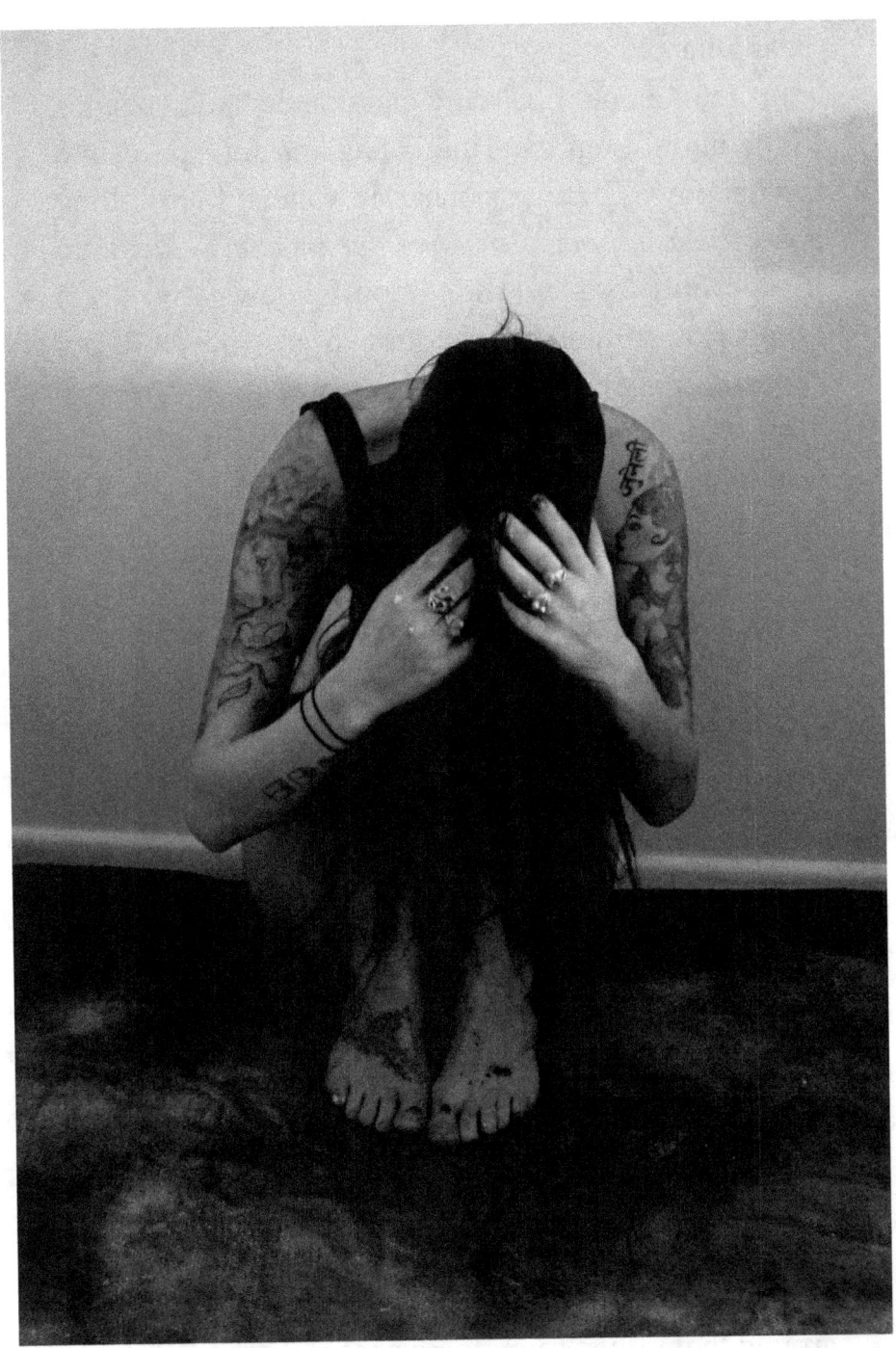

Dear Diary,

I am alone. I pass my classmates like two ships in the night. I am the Titanic heading full speed into the unknown. I am in uncharted waters. I am falling apart. *Please, I beg. Someone get me some glue.* I am irretrievably broken and I don't know why. I am lying on the floor of my dorm room shower. I am covered in my own vomit. I am a mess.

The feeling of something not being right is becoming overwhelming. My thoughts are running wild and it feels like someone else is inside my head, in control of my body. *I can't be going insane! Mental illness runs in the family! How could this happen to me? What will people think? Will they believe I am crazy or that I lost it? I don't know what is wrong. I am not myself. I am someone else. But who? Who is this person I have become?*

I have been putting up a super brave front. I have been hiding the extent of my pain. I am mourning the loss of a dear loved one. But something else is wrong. I cry a lot and when I am not crying, I wish I was. I am here and I am not. I am distant and I am close. My life is a mixture of hyperbolic paradoxes. I don't sleep and I barely eat. I am too anxious and jittery to be around anyone else.

I can't sit with my friends in the cafeteria. I can't walk with them to class. Whenever I am around them I just seem to be absent. I see them look at me. I see them wondering what is going on in my head as I stare off blankly into space. But I can't seem to break my trance. As the days go on, I lose the energy to fake engagement in their conversations. How can I talk about such trivial things when my world is falling apart?

I don't give a shit what you wear to the next party! I don't care what boy you currently have a crush on and I don't care about our upcoming contracts exam! I want to turn back the clock. I want to reverse time and go back to a few months ago when everything was fine. I want to be just a normal girl at university whose greatest concern is the lack of variation in the cafeteria menu. I want to be as carefree as I once was.

None of this feels real. It is all too much. I can't think about anything else right now except for the loss of my mum. Yet I also don't feel like I have a right to be upset. But at the same time, I feel like I should be more upset. How can I move on when she is gone? I can't let this grief go. I cannot switch it off. I can't simply push it to the side and study. The only time I can forget about it is when I am drunk. So I drink. I drink when I wake up, I drink every time I return to my dorm room. I drink all night until I pass out. I drink until I turn my insides out. I drink until the uncomfortable feeling is gone.

I run for hours each and every day. I physically

can't stop. I have lost weight. I am really thin. I don't care how I look. Right now I don't really care about much except making all of this go away. I wish I could forget any of this ever happened. I am lost. I have no one to grieve with. The uni campus is full of students, but I am still alone. I am by myself in a sea of people. I wake up each day and just see a video montage of my life. Everything is a blur. It's like a movie scene where I stand still and the rest of the world passes by in fast forward.

I am failing my classes. I can't think, I can't study and I can't prepare. I know the wheels are falling off my wagon. I am slowly sinking in this quicksand. I don't even know any more if I want to be helped. Am I too far gone? Is this really what my life has become? I don't want to be the captain that goes down with this ship. *Help. I see no other way out.*

Captain Barbie

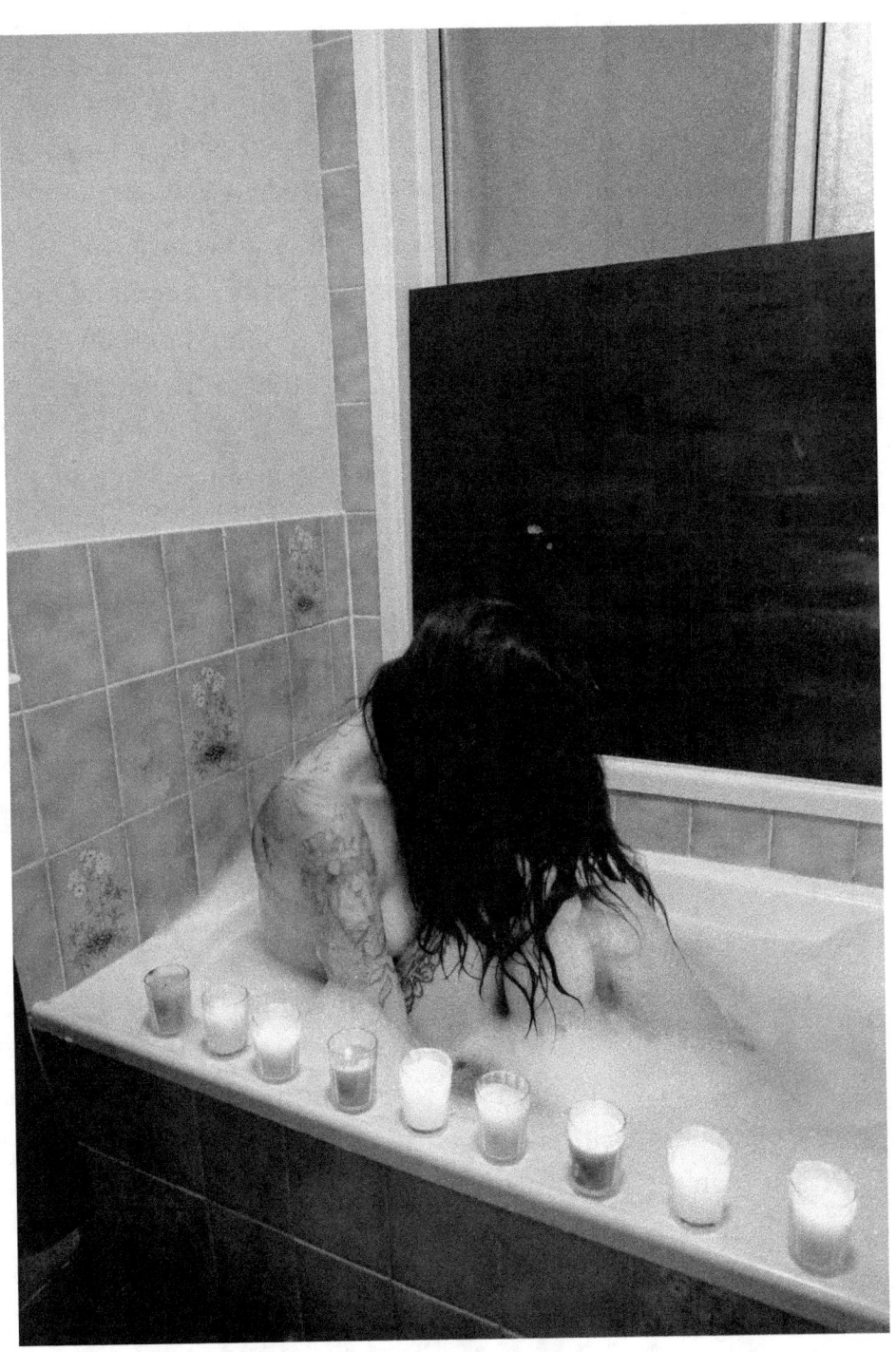

Dear Diary,

I am not in control of my mind. Who is creating these horrible thoughts in my head? Where did they come from and why are they here?

It's like a different DJ has taken over my own personal radio station. The transmission is mixed. The show must go on, but I wake the next day feeling worse than I did before. But that is the nature of the beast. It seems to drag on and on. First it took control of me, then it sucked the life from me. Now it's devouring me whole and spitting my rotten corpse back out.

I used to be the life of the party, but now that the fire inside me has been put out, I'm not that fun to be around. I wish I was; I really do. But without drugs or alcohol I can't fight what's in my head. I need something to lift me up. Boost me up so I can float on the surface of this vast darkness I'm drowning in. Please don't shame me for no longer wanting to swim.

I can't seem to find a reason to laugh or smile, or even a reason to cry. There's no reason to live and my only reason to die is to rid my body and mind of the pain in which I slowly suffocate. I can't sleep but I also can't get out of my bed. The only time I leave is when I am in so much pain I flop into the bathtub. I let the water run over me and sink below the surface just to test the waters, I want to know what it would feel like to stay there forever. I imagine the vast ocean that has become my life. Dark, deep and lonely. There's solace in my isolation but the constant state of melancholy is nothing like the wonderful life I was promised. Only two things are certain. I know what's below me (the bottom of the ocean) and what's above (the sky), but going down just means you will certainly die, and there's no chance of going up! My options are limited and slim.

Others don't believe me. I can see them, but they can't see me. I see my friends and family in boats just out of my reach. I'm screaming out to them for help, but no one seems to hear.

"Just throw a life buoy," I scream. "Just give me a rope! Pull me to safety," I urge. But no one is moving. I scream louder with panic, and try to swim towards them, but they are infuriatingly always just out of reach. It's a terrifying and frustrating feeling to have everyone you know watching your struggle, but no one lending a hand. I don't understand why they won't save me. No one even tries. It would be so simple, but they act as if they don't know how. It's like they are too scared to approach me, so they keep their distance. What are they so afraid of? Mental illness is not contagious!

Sometimes, I just get so exhausted from treading water and screaming for help, that I just stop and begin sinking. I hold my breath for what feels like forever and prepare to meet death. I wait for the inevitable end to the permanent war of struggles in my head. But for some strange reason, every time I disappear beneath the surface, that last surge of energy and motivation strikes. I really want to give up, but my body won't let me; like no matter how much my mind wants me to die, my body does not. A primitive instinct for survival kicks in, and I burst through the surface of the water and take a big breath of fresh air. Sometimes, that's all it takes. I don't know why I'm still here or what drove me to so desperately latch on to hope. Even when it didn't look like it was there. I have learnt to accept disappointment but never lose hope. It's not that I have faith things will work out, because faith believes in the unbelievable. Hope to me is different. Hope means going on when everything seems so pointless. I have learnt to have faith that when everything seems like it is falling apart, it may just be falling into place. I believe that HOPE is an acronym for Hold On, Pain Ends. It is not my suffering and hurt that I want to shape my future. I believe that everything happens for a reason. I wish I knew that reason, but I don't just yet. I don't know why I strongly believe that just because things are not happening for me right now doesn't mean they never will. I have every reason to lose hope, but then

I will feel helpless. Helplessness is the true definition of the last point before giving up. I try to stay as far away from that line as possible because crossing it only leads to one thing.

I wonder why I am attracted to water. Is it because I am a cancer? A crab? I know water is a symbol of our emotions and perhaps the recurring theme of drowning in a body of water simply means I am drowning in my emotions. They say dreaming about drowning can be provoked by repressed emotions. I wonder if daydreams count. I have a lot of those. It could also mean that I am over doing something. I seem to be over doing everything except living. Being overwhelmed by my sheer existence is just the norm for me. Maybe my subconscious is painting an un-pretty picture. Apparently dreaming of drowning can be a serious warning too. I feel like I am dying. I am not living life on the safe side. I am reckless. I live with no regard for self-preservation.

Sometimes, I look at myself in the mirror and see a complete stranger staring back at me. She is so different from how I see myself. Whenever I imagine myself in my mind, the real version of me, she is screaming under water. My spirit is trapped in some sort of sack of fluid. She can't get out, like a premature baby unable to escape the embryo sack. I make a lot of noise, but cannot be heard. I hope that perhaps I am heading for a sort of baptism. I would do anything for a do-over. I wish I could be reborn. I want to hit restart. Life seems to end when you are overwhelmed by depression and sorrow. I would do anything to feel alive once more.

    I am afraid of being like this for the rest of my life. Hope to me is the only thing stronger than fear. It is what allows me to push through the fear so that I have a chance at a better life. Failure is not an option. I will never settle. There are two types of giving up, and one certainly is not an option for me. Giving up isn't just about committing suicide, you can give up fighting without ending it. The saddest fate I could ever meet is to stop trying to get better. Even if this illness doesn't kill me, it will certainly rob me of my life. I am not okay with that. I hate thieves. I will not let it steal my life out from underneath my feet. I will not let it take away all the happiness this life has to offer.

Tin Man Barbie

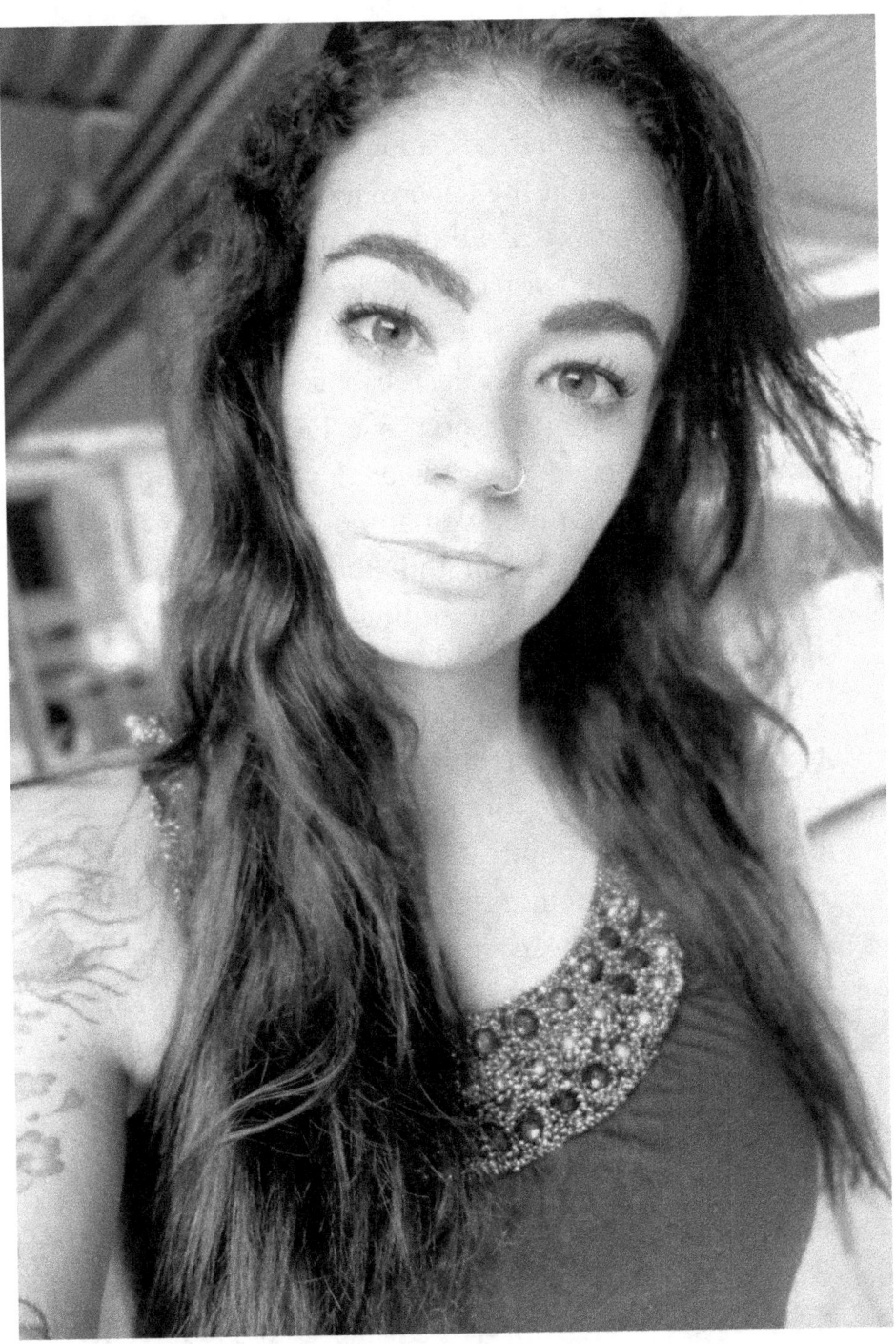

Dear Diary,

My mother called me today. I wasn't feeling well. I listened to her talk about the town gossip and what she bought at the supermarket with this absurd demeanour that it was all important information, but really I knew it wasn't worth anything much more than being discarded like those unwanted purchases in the closet from her last trip to the shops. She persisted in telling me how she had vacuumed the house and cleaned the shower. I was listening and thinking, how can this woman believe any of this is important? Here I am on the balcony of my apartment leaning on the railing wondering if it was high enough to jump. Would three floors be enough?

I thought about the perfect drop and me falling to my death. I could feel it, the air rushing past, the weight of gravity forcing me down. It felt so liberating. I felt numb. Dead inside. I felt nothing though as I strained my neck over the edge, looking down at all of those students that were going by below. If I jumped, they would think that someone had been in some kind of accident or something terrible had happened on the balcony, but it wouldn't be true because what has happened in my head is much worse than anything else ever could be. I was in a terrible state and needed to make a decision. Despite the drop not being high enough, there was the possibility that since I lived on a busy university campus with high foot traffic that someone would find me and call an ambulance.

After about half an hour she finally paused, took a breath and asked me how I was doing. I didn't have time for her nonsense anymore. I was over sugar coating things. I had been allowing her to live in blissful ignorance for long enough.

"I'm not doing too well," I replied.

"Why?" She asked, surprised.

"I don't know …" I trailed off. "I don't feel okay. I feel depressed, like I don't want to live any more. Nothing brings me joy. I'm not living. I only exist, barely surviving." I finally admitted.

There was a pause.

"I don't want to hear that!" she giggled.

"Well, I don't want to be like this!" I cried.

"Oh, don't be a drama queen," she joked.

There was an awkward pause before she warned "Don't call me again unless you have something positive to say."

Did I need to remind her that she had called me?

Frustrated, I hung up. I sighed. My heart was broken. *It is official, no one cares about me.*

I feel bad about hanging up on my mum. She'd sounded really hurt by the way I had said it. But when she asked me how I was, why was there a big silence? Well that's because the thought of continuing the long drawn out conversation with her sent chills down my spine. All she ever does is talk and talk. She never listens to anything anyone else has to say or think for themselves. This is why things end badly between us every time we speak; she always finds something wrong with what I say and argues against me until I get so frustrated that even if it starts out as a small disagreement, somehow it escalates into an all-out war.

Disheartened Barbie

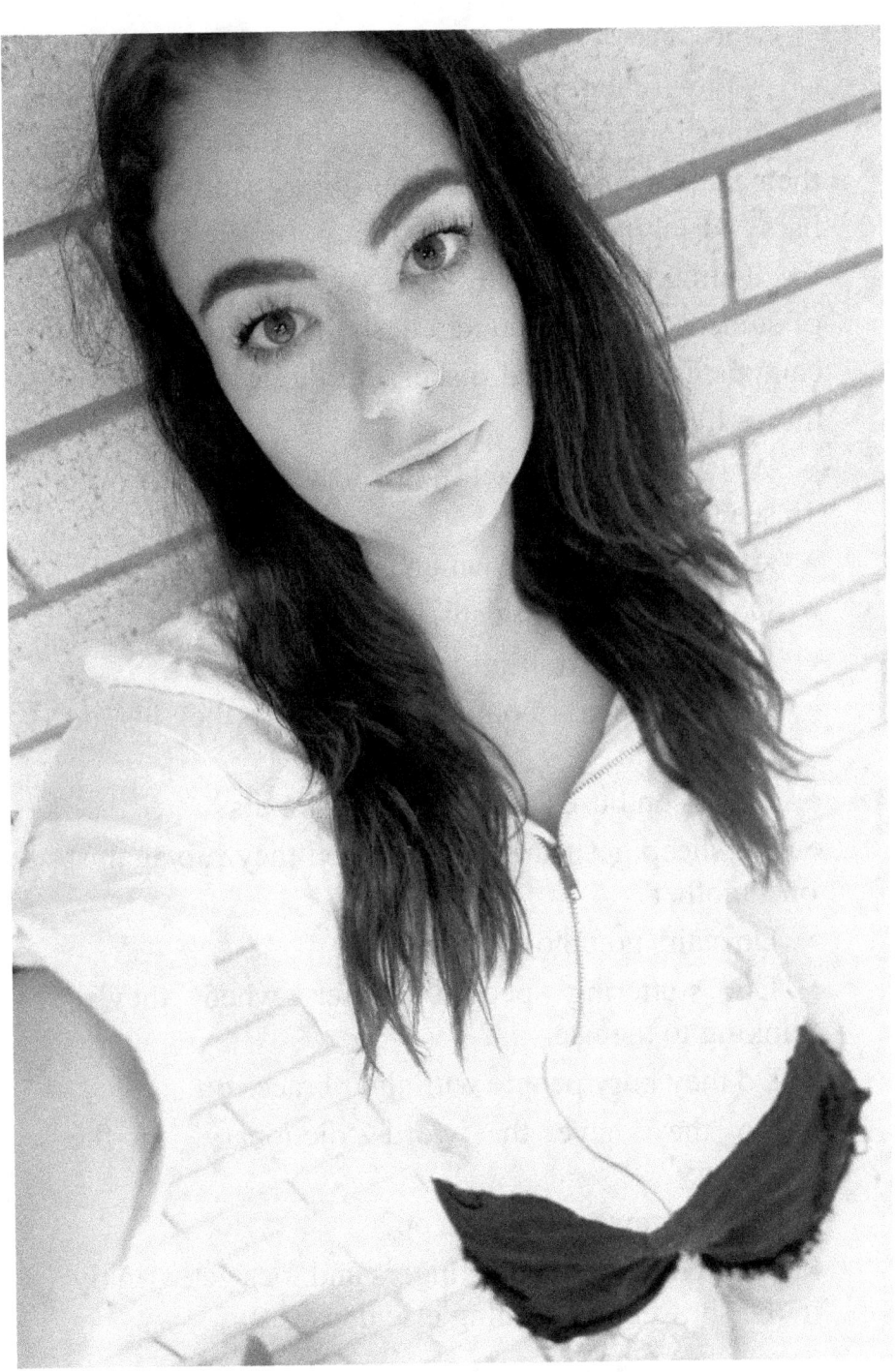

Dear Diary,

Law school is the kind of place you can ask the big questions in life. You will often find students in their natural habitat, either the library study, the uni bars drinking and discussing irrelevant yet fascinating trivia. At any time you will find a bunch of students sitting around a desk, devouring some on campus cafeteria food discussing thought provoking things like:

- Are children who act in rated 'R' movies allowed to see them?
- At a movie theater, which arm rest is yours?
- Do animals commit suicide?
- Do coffins have lifetime guarantees?
- Do dentists go to other dentists or do they just do it themselves?
- Do prison buses have emergency exits?
- Do sheep get 'static cling' when they rub against one another?
- Do stairs go up or down?
- Do stuttering people stutter when they're thinking to themselves?
- Do they bury people with their braces on?
- Do they have the word 'dictionary' in the dictionary?
- Do you yawn in your sleep?
- How come only your fingers and toes get wrinkly in the shower and nothing else does?

- How come you never see a billboard being put up by the highway? It always seems to just be there...
- How far east can you go before you're heading west?
- If a baby's leg pops out at 11:59PM but his head doesn't come out until 12:01, which day was he born on?
- If a doctor suddenly had a heart attack while doing surgery, would the other doctors work on the doctor or the patient?
- If a guy that was about to die in the electric chair had a heart attack would they save him?
- If a kid refuses to sleep during nap time, are they guilty of resisting a rest'?
- If a pack of gum says that each piece is 10 calories, is that amount just chewing the gum, or also for swallowing it?
- How many people swallow gum and does it really take 10 years to digest?
- If an ambulance is on its way to save someone, and it runs someone over, does it stop to help them?
- If parents say, "Never take candy from strangers" then why do we celebrate Halloween?
- If the sky's the limit, then what is space, *over the limit*?
- If you blew a bubble in space would it pop?
- If you dug a hole through the center of the earth, and jumped in, would you stay at the center because of gravity?

◆ If you try to fail, and succeed, which have you done?

◆ Is it possible to be allergic to water? Yes and it's called *Aquagenic Urticaria.*

◆ Is there a time limit on fortune cookie predictions?

◆ Since bread is square, then why is sandwich meat round?

◆ What do you do when you see an endangered animal that is eating an endangered plant?

◆ What is another word for 'thesaurus'?

◆ What would happen to the sea's water level if every boat in the world was taken out of the water at the same time?

◆ What's the difference between normal ketchup and fancy ketchup?

◆ When does it stop being partly cloudy and start being partly sunny?

◆ When French people swear, do they say 'pardon my English'?

◆ Why are the little styrofoam pieces called peanuts? How many people have tried to sue packing companies thinking they were edible?

◆ Why are there interstate highways in Hawaii?

◆ Why do they say a football team is the 'world champion' when they don't play anybody outside the US?

◆ Why does grape flavor smell the way it does when actual grapes don't taste or smell anything like that?

- Why does the Easter bunny carry eggs? Rabbits don't lay eggs.
- Why doesn't *McDonald's* sell hot dogs? Apparently the founder Ray Kroc had prohibited the company from selling hot dogs because he said there is no telling what is inside hot dog meat. As opposed to any other mcdonalds meat? Apparently Americans consume around 150 million hot dogs on 4th of July each year.
- Why don't the hairs on your arms get split ends?
- Why is it that on a phone or calculator the number five has a little dot on it?
- Why is the Lone Ranger called 'Lone' if he always has his Indian friend Tonto with him?
- Why is there a light in the fridge and not in the freezer?
- Why is vanilla ice cream white when vanilla extract is brown?

It blows my mind how many people in law school actually know the answers to some of these nonsensical trivia questions. I guess because we sit around all day bothering to ask them. There is a whole category of genius for people who know the most obscure and insanely irrelevant facts. The kind of people that tell you most toilets flush in the note of E flat. That Cap'n Crunch's full name is Horatio Magellan Crunch. I guess it's helpful if you ever wanted to go on a trivia winning streak.

I have learnt some fascinating although totally

useless things today:

◆ At any one time about 0.7% of the world's population is drunk.

◆ The Vatican City is the country that drinks the most wine per capita at 74 litres per citizen per year.

◆ 315 entries in *Webster's Dictionary* were misspelled.

◆ For every non-porn webpage, there are five porn pages.

◆ Grapes explode when you put them in the microwave. Wait a minute, I actually do need to try this one. Brb.

◆ King Henry VIII slept with a gigantic axe beside him. Just in case he had to behead another wife I guess. He also had a 'Groom of the Stool': whose job was to monitor and assist in the King's bowel movements. The role remained in existence until King Edward VII abolished it in 1901.

◆ Approximately 40,000 Americans are injured by toilets each year.

◆ If a female ferret does not have sex for a year, she will die. Personally I think this a fact made up by a bunch of teenage ferret boys trying to scare their girlfriends into having sex with them regularly. Just like when my housemate convinced her live-in boyfriend that she had to wear underpants at night because otherwise spiders can crawl up into your vagina while you sleep. I guess he was willing to risk his butthole becoming a spider's den then because he never seemed to wear pants in the bedroom. Fun Fact:

♦ Crocodile poop used to be used as contraception. Probably because no one wanted to stick their penis in a vagina full of shit.

♦ There are five calories in a teaspoon of semen. Although I am pretty sure every teenage boy will tell you the last one when they are trying to encourage you to give them head. *Ew!* Soz boys, I'm on a calorie restricted diet.

Cinema trivia is also quite common. Learning facts like: that

♦ Christian Bale reportedly studied Tom Cruise's mannerisms to prepare for his role as the serial killer in American Psycho.

♦ Sean Connery wore a toupee in all his James Bond movies.

♦ Nicholas Cage bought a pet octopus once because he sincerely thought it might help with his acting.

♦ Nicholas Cage also once did magic mushrooms with his cat.

We know from our legal studies that cocaine used to be advertised to be used for a wide range of things including relief from toothaches and headaches. Heroin was advertised as an alternative to aspirin. I don't know why it surprised me when I was informed that Ketchup was sold in the 1830s as medicine too.

I am now privy to some pointless facts like

'almost' is the longest word in English with all the letters in alphabetical order.
- It actually takes 142.18 licks to reach the center of a Tootsie pop.
- 1% of all women can achieve full orgasm just by stimulating their breasts.
- You'll eat more than 35,000 cookies in your lifetime (probably).
- Steve Jobs relieved stress by soaking his feet in Apple's company toilets. Now that is just fucked up!
- Fredric Baur was the man who invented the iconic *Pringles* can. When he died, his ashes were buried in one.
- Homosexuality was still classified as an illness in Sweden in 1979. Swedes responded by calling into work 'sick', saying they 'felt gay'.
- There is enough sperm in one single man to impregnate every woman on earth. So why cant one man just give a baby to every woman who wants one and the rest of us will never have to have sex again?
- It is impossible to sneeze with your eyes open.
- There is a town in Canada called 'Dildo'.
- Human birth control pills work on gorillas.
- France was still executing people by guillotine when the first Star Wars movie came out.
- All swans in England belong to the queen.
- No piece of square paper can be folded more than 7 times in half.

- The US Treasury once considered producing doughnut-shaped coins!
- It's been said that nearly 3% of the ice in Antarctic glaciers is penguin urine.
- The hashtag symbol is technically called an octothorpe.
- There is a Boring, Oregon and a Dull, Scotland. They have been sister cities since 2012.
- At the 1908 Olympics, the Russians showed up 12 days late because they were using the Julian calendar instead of the Gregorian calendar.
- The Kola Superdeep Borehole in Russia is the world's deepest hole. It is 7.5 miles deep, but interestingly, only 9 inches wide. Perhaps they tried to tunnel their way through until they realised they couldn't fit through the hole.
- Serial killer Ted Bundy once received a commendation from the Seattle Police Department for chasing down a purse snatcher.
- Lord Byron allegedly kept a pet bear in his dorm room while studying at Cambridge University.
- A group of flamingos is called a 'flamboyance'.

Whoever said procrastination was unproductive never spent time in a law library.

Thought Provoking Barbie

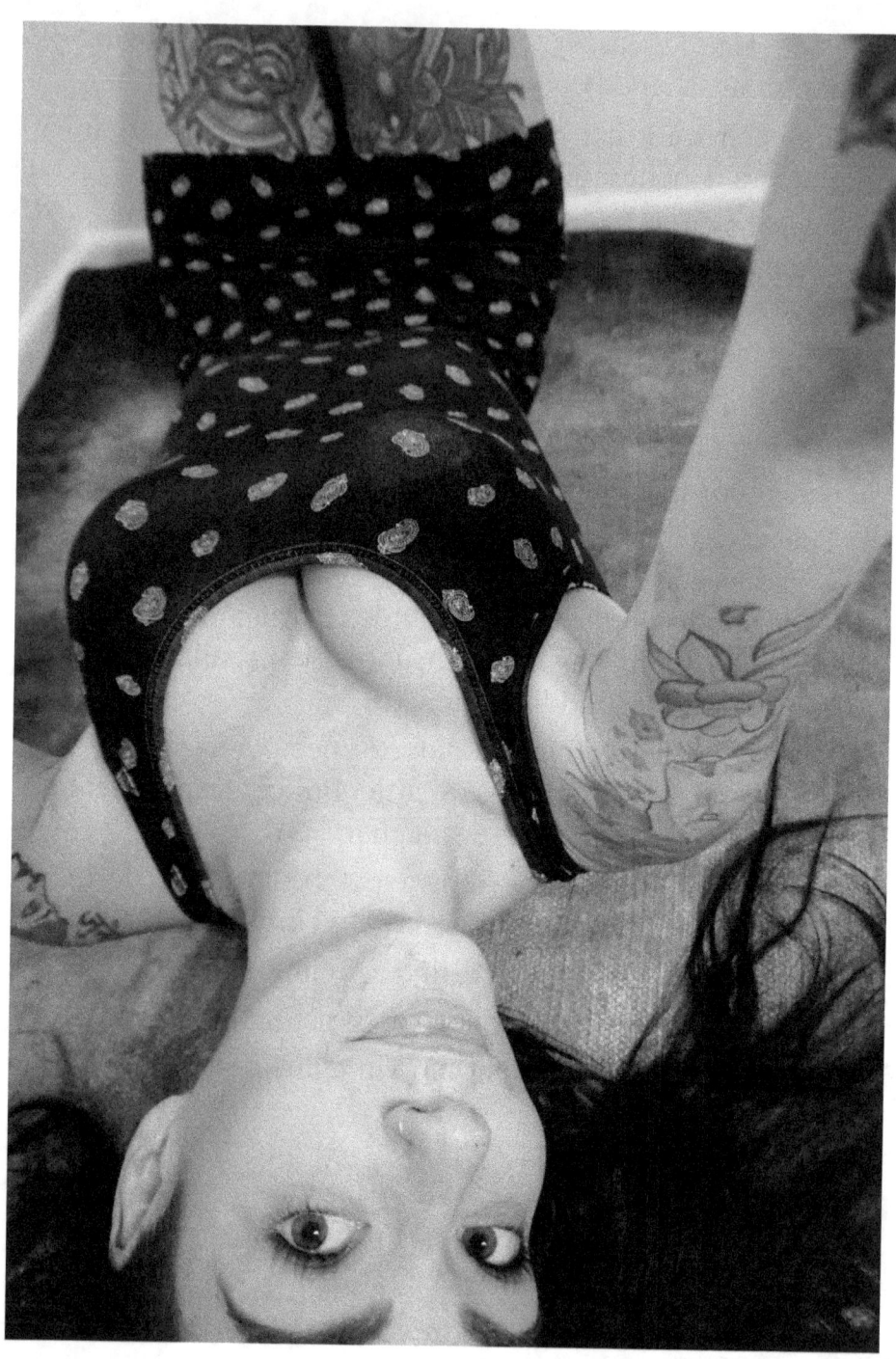

Dear Diary,

I sat in class today, a two-hour Land Law lecture on Native Title and the case of Mabo. I really tried to be present. I tried to focus, but my mind was running wild, like stallions in the Snowy Mountains. I was burning up despite the intense, cool breeze coming from the ice-cold industrial air conditioning system. My body twitched, and my legs bounced up and down, like a clown on a pogo stick. I felt claustrophobic in this huge lecture theatre.

My heart was racing and my mouth was dry. The lights were dimmed so I could only barely see the outline of the professor at the podium. Unable to recall all that I had tried so hard to commit to memory, panic set in quickly.

The professor's voice boomed across the room, like a god thundering down from the heavens. The clicks of the slide changer were like nails down a chalkboard. The squeak of the whiteboard marker sounded like he was carving Egyptian hieroglyphs into the Pyramids.

It was like my mind was highlighting the most insignificant of sounds. The tiers in this room reminded me of a Greek amphitheatre. The sound bounced off the walls and echoed like a rap track doused with reverb. The sound of students smashing their fingers against the keys of their laptops was like a stadium applauding their favourite team's goal.

I felt like I was in a Roman gladiator arena. The crowd cheered! But when I looked around, no one was making a sound.

I imagined it as the soundtrack that the man in front of me must have muted on his computer, as I could see from behind that he had nothing but a Canadian hockey team's latest game playing on his screen.

Suddenly my heart started pounding against my ribcage like a caged animal trying to escape. My breath became shorter, and I was sure I was about to explode with rage. *Rage?* What the hell for? I was filled with adrenaline ready to run. But from what? There was no threat lurking in this classroom. Or was there? Which one of my fellow classmates was the psychopath hiding in our midst? Was it one of the 'cool' boys hiding in the back row gawking at pictures of hot chicks? Was it one of the most diligent students in the front row? Was it the guy dressed in Ralph Lauren?

Wow, that escalated quickly!

One minute I was following Mabo vs Queensland and Eddie's bid. The next I was halfway down Dante's Inferno Pit as paranoia set in.

I lasted about 15 minutes in that room, before I packed my notebook into my bag and made a run for the exit. I sprinted up the stairs, for the first time in my life not scared of face planting on the step.

I ignored the concerned faces of my friends as I exited the room. I didn't stop running; I just ran for four hours straight. I got home and did push ups, squats and jumped on the spot until I dropped. I had this nervous energy I just couldn't stop. I went straight to the shop and that was when I bought my first ever pack of cigarettes.

Just like that, life as I know it has stopped. Law school is never going to be the same. I have changed.

I don't know what was going on with me. I just want desperately to rest. Instead, I find myself in a state of desperate distress.

Manic Barbie

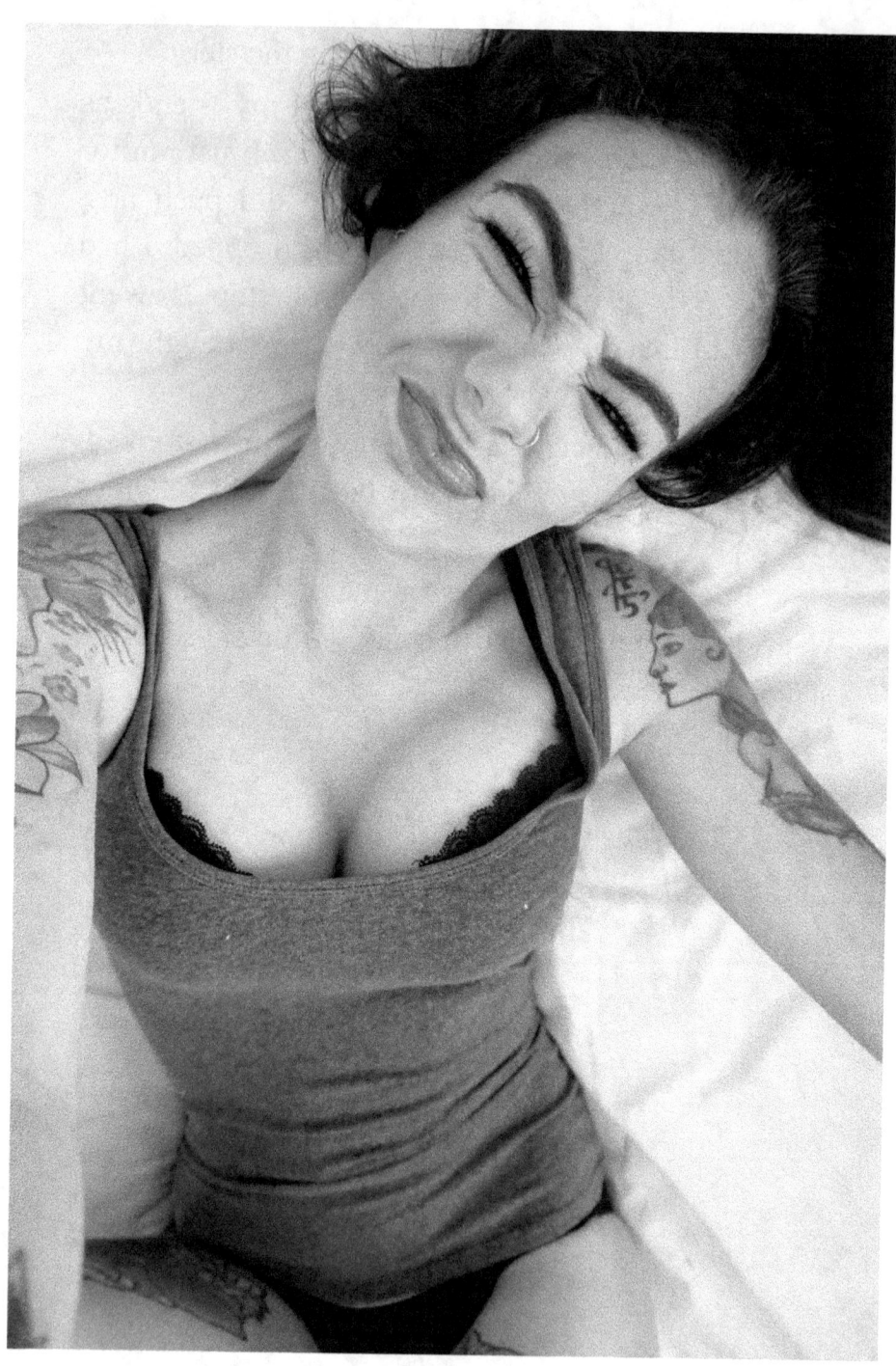

Dear Diary,

There are fireworks in my brain. Something is happening up in there. A storm is brewing. My head hurts. It is fizzing and bubbling like Coco Pops crackling in a cereal bowl. I pace around with my head in my hands. I lean up against the wall and tenderly bang my head against it. I pull back and throw my hands up in the air. I want to scream! But I return to my wall. I bounce my forehead against the brick. I wonder how much it would hurt if I just beat myself to death?

I want the race to halt. I want the clock to stop ticking and the screaming to subside. I pull back again and pace around my tiny dorm room. I jump up and down on the spot. I want to shake this tension in my body. I jump down to the floor and do one hundred sit ups. Then I squat. I work out for an hour just trying to tire myself out. My chest is getting tight and it's really hot. I have the aircon on full. It's like Antarctica here. I swear I just saw a penguin …

I want to go outside and go for a walk but its pitch black and all the shops are shut. I don't want to look like a deranged person running around the streets at 3am. I also don't want to meet an unhinged person alone on the streets at 3am. I don't want to be murdered or raped. I don't want to die but I also don't want to live, not like this. Not anymore.

For the first few nights in a row I am not

drunk. As the semester goes on the party life dwindles. Everyone else is getting serious about their assessments and exams. I am just over here, exhausted yet unable to sit still. I lay on my bed and stare at the ceiling. I have decorated it with a thousand fairy lights. I count the bulbs one by one like sheep, trying to fall asleep. It feels like an eternity has passed but it's probably only been a second. I spring back up and start to look at the photos I have posted on my wall. I run my fingers over the photos with love, until I see a picture of my long lost mum. I grip my fingers into a fist and once again against the wall I thud.

 I want to chuck a tantrum. I want to scream and beat the wall to a pulp until my knuckles bleed. I want to cause a scene. I want to wake everyone up. But I don't. That would not be kind or courteous of me. I am not that selfish. I am not worth the attention. What good would it do anyway? People would just want to fix me, but there is no fix for this.

 I text everyone I know asking if anyone is up. I check my phone. No one replies. I walk down my corridor and end up in the shower. I don't even bother to get undressed. I just step under the water fully clothed. Time is lost and then I am on the floor. I'm staring at the gap under the door. I use a shampoo bottle as a pillow so my ear doesn't lay on the floor of the communal showers. I am beyond the point of worrying how disgusting this is. It isn't my first rodeo. Every day I do the same thing. I don't plan to, but I really don't know what else to do with myself.

    First I try to find a distraction. I start off with my good friends and work my way down the list until I get to acquaintances and eventually pot heads I tolerate for the free weed. But no one is available tonight. I wonder if they know it could be my last one?

    I try to control my mind. It's not alright. A thousand words a second are sprinting across my brain. It's like a million trains at Grand Central Station. It is gridlocked. But there is also a magical system where things can just suddenly disappear into thin air and then nothing ever crashes. I can't keep track of the timetable because who the fuck even knows where the stations are? Why is there a unicorn driving the train?

Rapid Thoughts Barbie

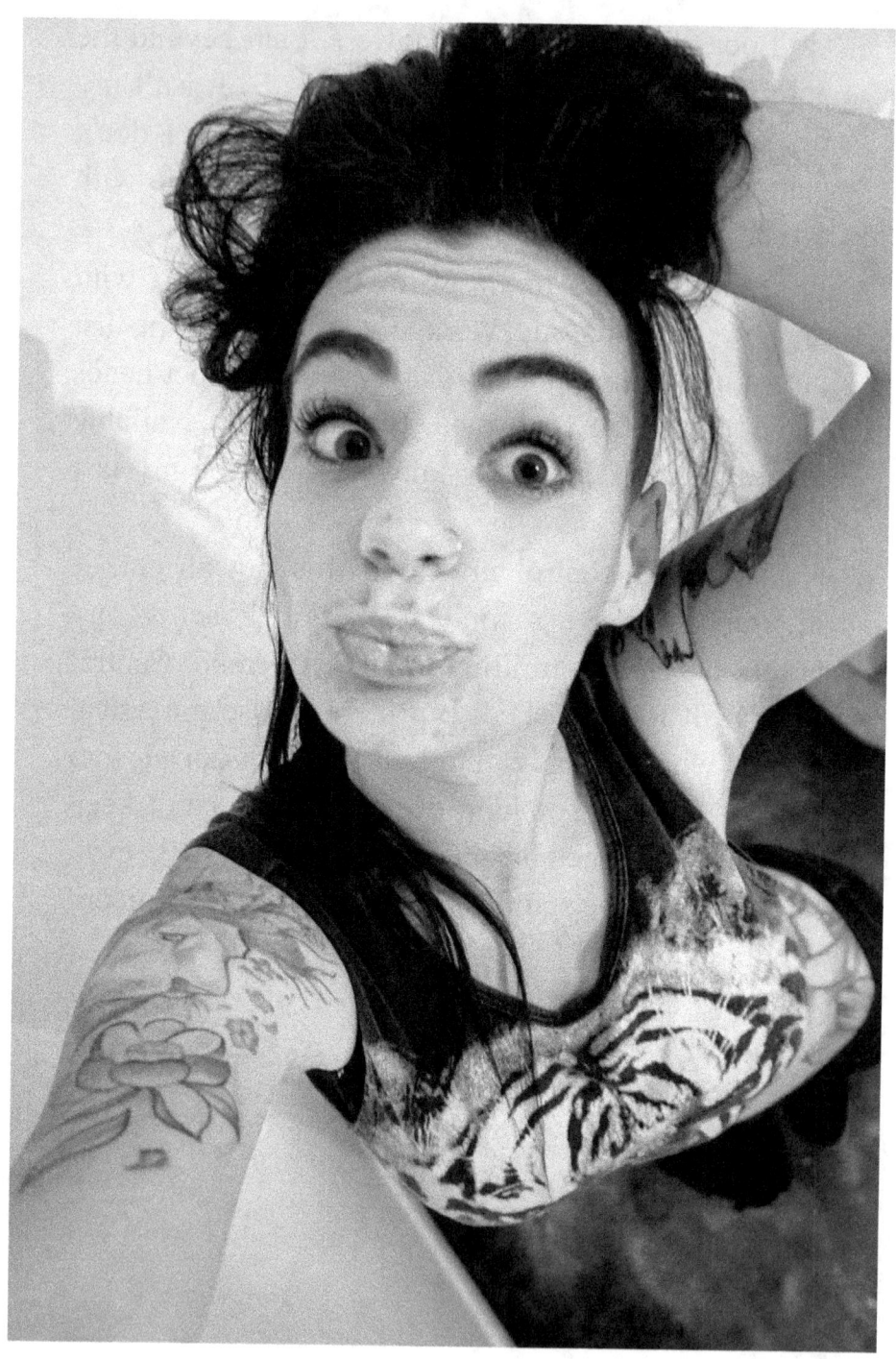

Dear Diary,

It is 2 am. Everyone else is asleep. The campus is dark. I am waiting for the gym to open up. I have been spending hours there every day. I work out because I am trying to burn all of this excess energy. Yet I walk out of the gym after two hours and run for another four. Then I have lunch and go back again that afternoon.

Everyone thinks I am just a dedicated 'fitness freak'. My girlfriends wish they had self-discipline like me. I don't think there is anything disciplined about it. It's more a form of self-destruction. I am slowly destroying my body. The more I work out the more body image issues I seem to develop. I pull at my skin in the mirror and post pictures of the skinny models I want to look like inside my wardrobe. I am jealous of my old self. I want to be the me that competed in the Miss universe pageant. I want to be that happy beautiful girl that had the world at her fingertips. I want to be anything other than what I am right now.

I am starving myself. It is really easy to do. I don't need to eat. In fact I *can't* eat. I find it hard to get anything down. My appetite is gone. I pretend like I have already gone to the cafeteria when others ask me to dinner. When I do go I eat a salad. I have been eating so much salad that I actually shit my pants today. It turns out a diet of only green veggies will give you extreme diarrhea. I was ready to walk into a Criminal Law lecture and felt it ooze out. I had to grab my jacket and tie it around my waist hoping no one would notice the growing stain on my pale blue tights.

I don't want to eat. I'm not hungry. Everything tastes horrible. I might as well be chewing cardboard. Eating is a chore. It tastes like nothing. Anything I do try to eat I have to choke down. It's like my stomach has shrunk. I find vegetables and watery foods more palatable. Carbs and protein are too heavy for me to digest. I can't eat more than a few bites before my stomach feels as though it is in knots and overworked. It hurts to swallow. I feel nauseous after eating just a little bit, let alone a meal.

Once I get back to my room I am angry with myself and disappointed so I collapse in bed. But I can't lay there long. I jump up again and pace around the room looking at all the art I have blue tacked to my dorm room wall. I scratch at my arms and chew the inside of my mouth. The world is vibrating around me. It's like I can see every individual atom.

I know my room is in a state of disarray, but I have no control over it. The thought of tidying it up never crosses my mind. And when it suddenly does, I am immediately overcome with a desire to run. I feel like I need to run. I need to get out of here. My heart rate increases and the world seems to be moving in slow motion. The walls start closing in around me and my chest is tightening as fast as it can possibly squeeze, compressing my lungs, suffocating me.

I quickly change my clothes into my gym gear as if it's a race against the clock. I am on a sinking ship; the Titanic and water is already breaching this floor. I grab my bag and head to the gym. I sprint there as if someone is hot on my tail. But it's crowded, too crowded, and I try to put blinkers on to avoid all the new friends this new sociable version of me has made.

Suddenly I regret all of the nights I spent being Chatty Cathy at all the parties this semester. Why did I have to be the life of the party? Why did I ever think being the centre of attention would be a good idea?

My friends wave at me from the treadmills and stationary bikes, I smile and wave slightly but keep walking to the weights section. I don't have the mental capacity to explain why I burst out of the lecture and never returned. At least in the weight section the boys talk a little less.

Fitness Barbie

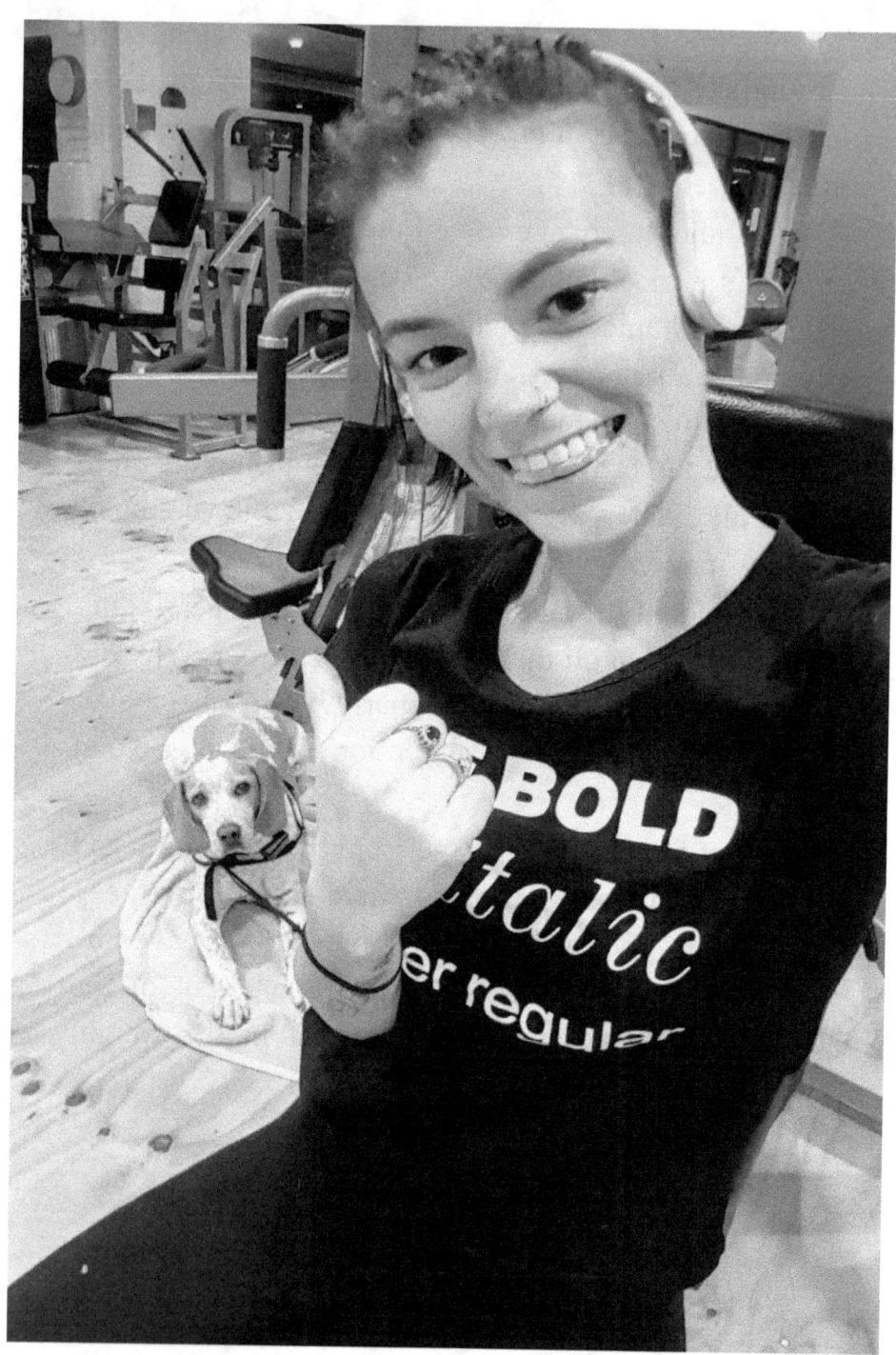

Dear Diary,

It's 5 am and my alarm is going off but I didn't get any sleep. I am sitting on the balcony of our common room watching the sunrise over the tall campus dorm buildings. The sun is just coming up over the courtyard trees, lighting up every window that faces out onto it with a beautiful light yellow glow. It is as if the world is dawning just for me.

Then it dawns on me. I have been up all night again. Smoking cigarettes like a steam train. I light up another one. There is something comforting about putting a cigarette in between your lips and cupping your hand around it while you light the end. The first puff is so satisfying. Unless your lighter doesn't work. Then absolute panic sets in. I can't say this cigarette is particularly wanted. My mouth is dry and burnt from the forty or so I've smoked all night.

I don't seem to get tired anymore. My mind is racing as idea after idea streams through my mind one after the next. Ideas of all the articles I could write for the student magazine. They seemed to like the last one my editor friend begged me to write late one night. Who knew I had a knack for writing?

I have been out here on the tiny balcony all night. It has become my little secret hiding place. I perch like a gargoyle over the courtyard watching students return to their rooms, so carefree in their ignorance. The campus is quiet at this time of the morning though. There are not many early risers at university. Except me, but my secret is to never sleep at all.

I listen to music and connect deeply with the song lyrics as they each begin to take on new meanings. Old songs played on repeat become anthems to my pain. New songs that I had never heard before become the soundtrack to my internal struggles. Sometimes music speaks so deeply to me it almost feels like a weapon – it cuts through my heart and dissects my soul with every note, chord progression or lyric in perfect time with the pain that is slicing through me.

My fingers find their way to my scalp as I scratch at my head trying not to think about all that is waiting for me today. The first day of classes seems like miles away but in reality, it's just another hour or two away from now. It's been so long since I've felt rested and cared for that these days are starting to blur together inside one big mess with no end in sight; one pattern repeating itself over and over again until nothing makes sense anymore. I am losing touch with reality.

Insomniac Barbie

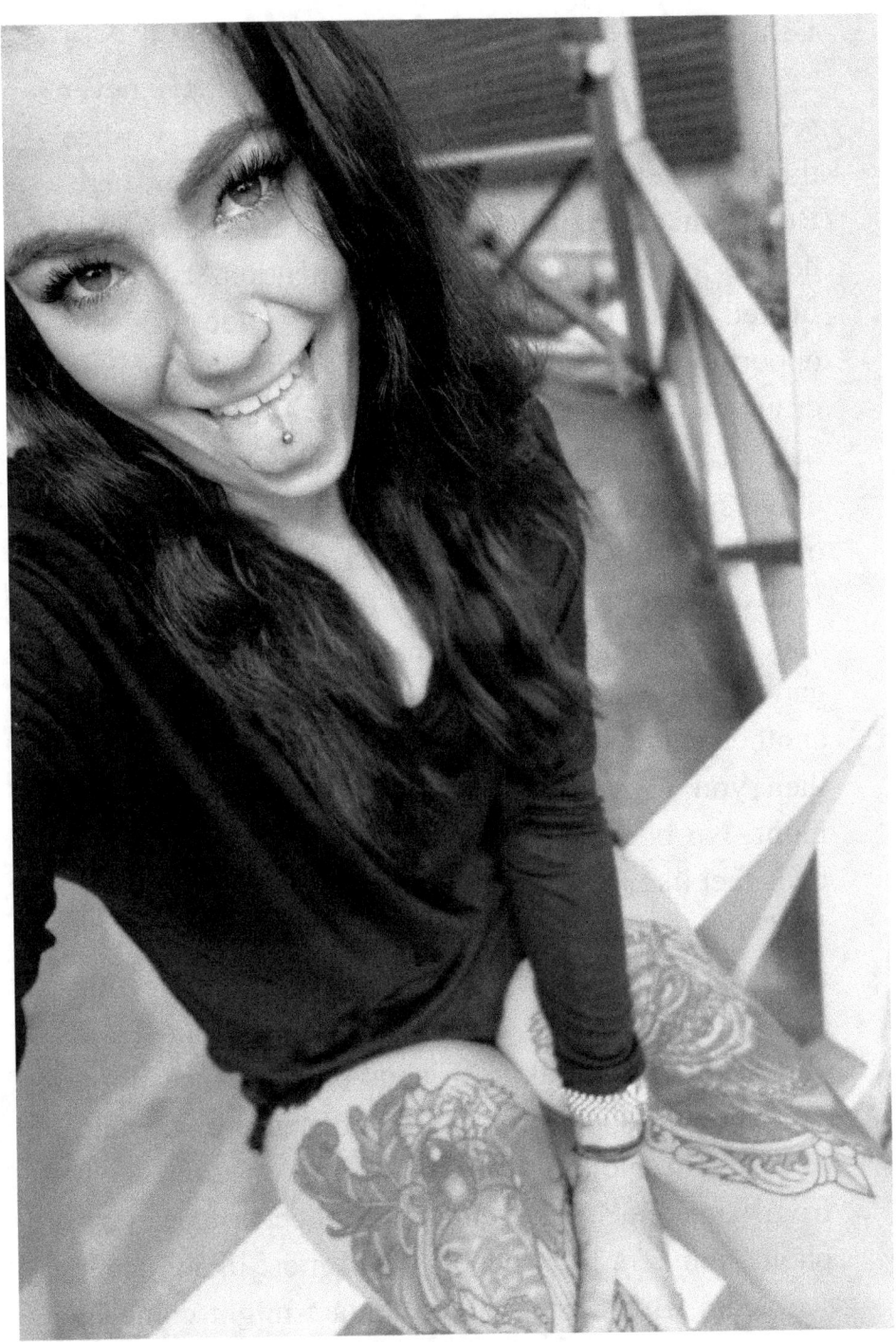

Dear Diary,

Someone said to me today that they have never seen me before, but have seen me every day since this semester started. Everyone thinks I am new here. But I am not. I just went from a bed-ridden quiet hermit to this manic centre of attention. I am too fucked up to be alone in my room. I look for any opportunity to socialise. I would rather be socially drunk than sober in my bed.

It is socially acceptable to be an alcoholic at university. Excessive drinking just seems to be part of the culture. You can get away with it if you just find a party to attend every day. The good thing about living on campus is that you do have a lot of gatherings to attend. Every night of the week there is another shindig. If you turn into a social butterfly, then you can hang with a different crowd every night. No one seems to get suspicious. Although it does feel like no one else drinks as much as me.

I have become rather good at going out by myself too. I have met so many new people this semester. Give me a little liquid courage and I am out on the town making friends on the dance floor. You know how it goes; we are old friends by the end of the night. Nothing says bonding like tequila shots from someone's belly button. I collect a variety of phone numbers from people I will most likely never see again. But perhaps their contact might come in handy should I need another excuse to drink.

    I have attended all of the university parties this semester. I am the life of the party. I am centre stage in every photograph. I am dancing on tables, tearing up the dance floor, doing jelly shots and living life for the party high. But when I get home after a night out, my mind returns to the place I left. I don't collapse in my bed too drunk to stand. I pace around and look for a distraction. The world around me spins. I seem to be gravitating to the floor so I slide down onto the carpet wriggling around like a worm trying to dig its way under the surface. I pass out for a moment but reality wakes me back up like a slap in the face. A shocking reminder that I am still alive.

    Life seems to be devoid of all meaning but in this state I don't really care. My face is numb and I giggle to myself as I roll around on the carpet. It smells, probably from the dried vomit I left there yesterday. Suddenly I get a strange wave of déjà vu. I have been here before. Alone in my room at 3am, just me and my thoughts.

    Sometimes I draw. I find it is the only way I can express what is going on inside my head. I will draw three or four pictures a night. For the first time in my life I am drawing pictures of girls. Up until now I was never very good at drawing people. I can't say I am much better, but I need to get these sketches out. I am reminded of a quote by Frida Kahlo "I never paint dreams or nightmares. I paint my own reality." Her paintings are a diary of her life, just as mine are. They adorn my walls. Some are falling off but I give each piece a stern talking to as I reattach them to the wall, demanding that they stay stuck.

There are really no words to describe the extent of what I feel right now. So I am having another drink. Tears are leaking out from my eyes as I try to shake away what has become a routine these past few months. I am choking on the taste of stale cans of alcohol. They are so strong and remind me of yesterday when I vomited the nasty liquid up. I don't know how much more I can have before my stomach ulcers flare up. In another wise quote from Frida, she said, "I tried to drown my sorrows, but the bastards learned how to swim".

That's pretty much where I am at all the time these days.

Alcoholic Barbie

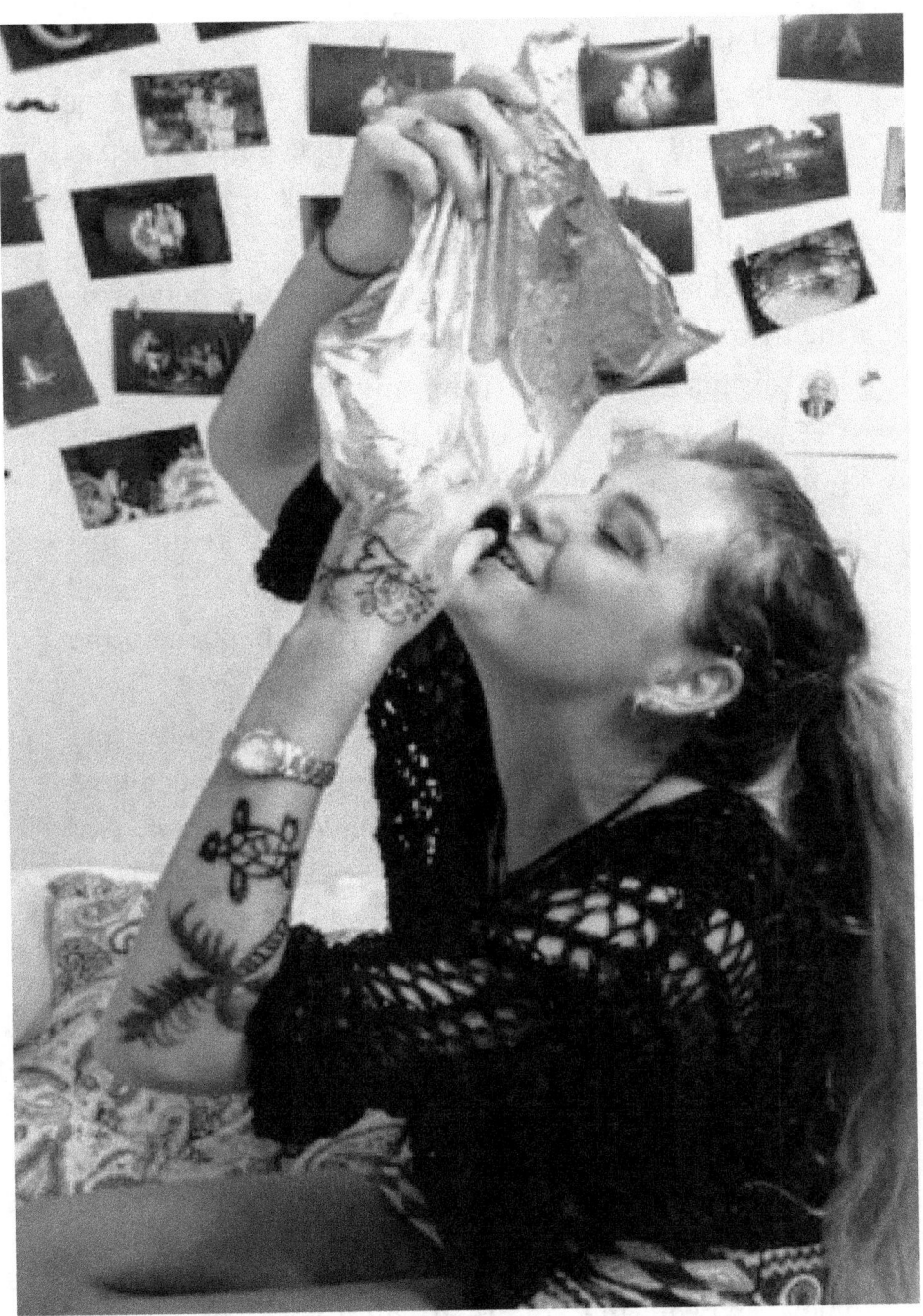

Dear Diary,

I can't keep track of who I am right now. One second I am laying on the floor like a dead corpse, the next I am dancing on a stripper pole in a packed nightclub, and then the next I am at work managing the hotel's front desk. One minute I am pondering the meaning of death and the next I am high on life. I am distancing myself from my feelings. Yet they overwhelm me still. I can't keep up with all that is going on. I just don't know what is wrong.

Is this really just grief? Am I really just depressed? Is this all I have left? When will it end? How will it end? Why did it have to happen in the first place? Why does everyone just keep encouraging me to move on? How can I move on? How can I simply study a law degree and act like I am not dead on the inside? I have told all of my teachers and professors what is going on. They know. To their credit the University has been very understanding. I am still failing though. No matter what personal tragedy I face, I am still expected to pass so that I can graduate.

This semester is going so fast. I doubt I will manage to get the marks to pass. I was doing so well before all of this happened. I was top of my class. I studied hard. Now I can't even read a paragraph. They expect me to read all these prescribed textbooks, case studies and judgements. The words just get muddled up on the page. I try to highlight what I write in the hopes it will help me focus. It doesn't help much. I just end up with a colourful page as incomprehensible as it was before.

My friends are trying to support me and help me the best they can. They *are* very supportive. But they just can't help me. I don't want to be alone. But they have class and they need to sleep. I *can't* sleep. I try to distract myself with people and parties, but there is only so much that goes on. I haven't slept for days. I don't remember the last time my eyes were closed. I am wide awake, pacing around my corridor. I am sitting on the balcony smoking a pack of cigarettes. I listen to music and chain smoke because I don't know what else to do.

Chain Smoker Barbie

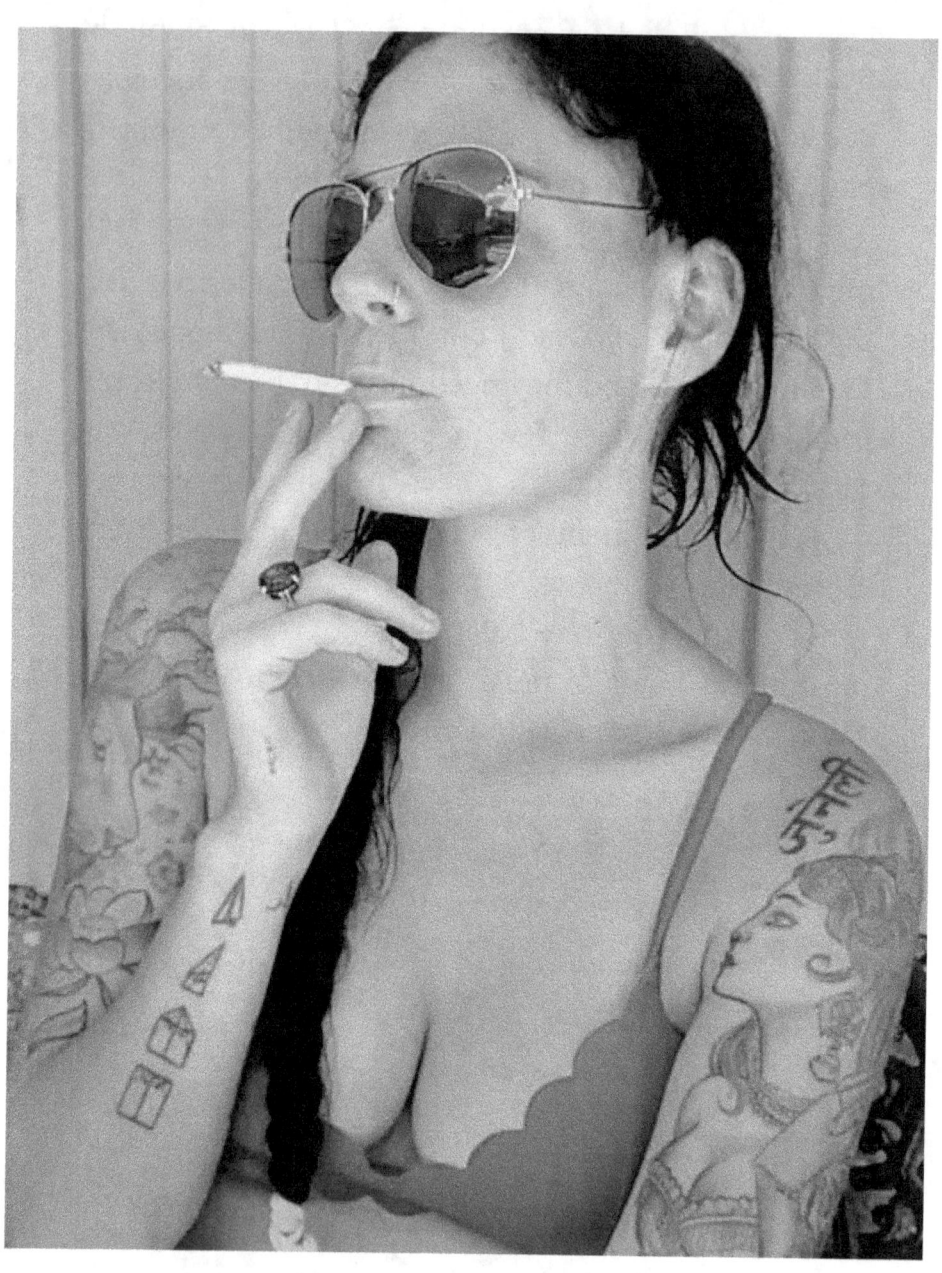

Dear Diary,

I'm still shaking, my hands are wet with sweat. There's a tremor in my bones, and the ground is unsteady beneath me. It hurts to breathe. The anxiety settles into my chest like an anchor weighing down half of me. My heart pounds faster and more erratically the closer I get to my dorm. I am almost running now, trying to shake this feeling off but it only seems to intensify as I near the entrance.

"Are you alright? Can I help you?" A student asks from her place on a bench outside the building. Her voice is soft and caring, but she doesn't understand that there's no helping me right now, not when I don't know what is going on. I can't breathe. My chest is being compressed. I am scared I can't get enough air into my lungs. I feel like I am having an asthma attack. But my puffer isn't helping.

Adrenalin is spreading through my body energizing every cell and synapse. It's like the sunlight is pouring into me and acting like radiation. It is illuminating every molecule in my organism like a bacterium attacking its host. I feel like I am transitioning into something that isn't human.

I thought things were bad in the lecture theatre but things are getting worse by the second. The leaves are sparkling. The sky is getting brighter. The landscape is illuminated with each object surrounded by a luminescent glow. I have never experienced anything like this. My eyes are fuzzy but my vision is super clear. The leaves, the sky, everything looks so beautiful and bright. There must be something in the air that makes everything seem more vibrant than usual.

My body feels electric. The adrenaline pumps through my veins and I feel like Superwoman; I can do anything. I burst through the doors of my dorm room and race to put on my running shoes. I speed back out and head down to the boardwalk. I run like Forrest Gump. I run until I can't anymore.

Eventually I get back to my dorm. Four hours have passed. Everyone else is getting ready for dinner but there is no way I can eat. I haven't had any appetite lately. Everything tastes like dirt. Maybe I am a vampire? That explains why I can't sleep at night.

The truth is, I don't know what I am. I am full of energy and my brain feels like it is on steroids. All my senses are enhanced. I am abnormally wired and extremely jumpy. I get up every two minutes to do a set of jumping jacks. I can't tell whether it is energy or agitation. Is there a difference? The ants in my pants want me to dance. So I jump up again and spin until I get giddy. I fall to the floor and laugh. About what, I don't know. Life just seems so magical. Yet mine also seems like a tragic fairy tale.

I am out onto the balcony and light up a

cigarette, listening to the same song on repeat. Save Tonight by Eagle Eye Cherry. I think it's such a sad song. Imagine if tonight was my last night? I do. I am imagining it over and over again. I imagine watching everyone react to my death. I wonder what they would think, feel and say.

Manic Barbie

I am drowning, but this sea isn't made of water, it consists of hopelessness, despair, guilt and shame.

Bipolar Barbie

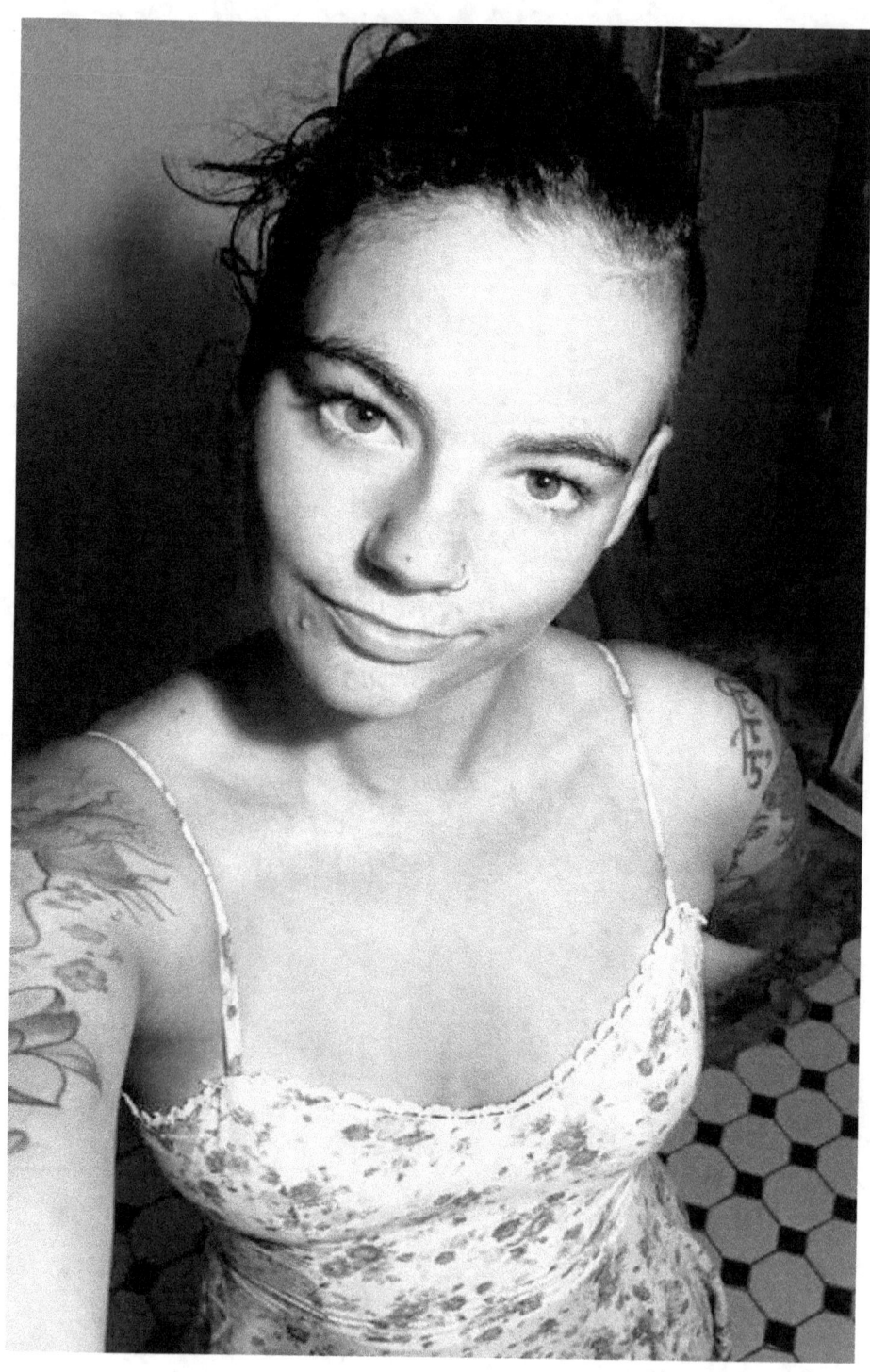

Dear Diary,

I just can't think. My brain is my superpower. My mind is my guide. Without it I have nothing. Have you ever tried to sit with a bunch of law students and keep up when your brain is concussed? I used to love our debates. I used to love our ridiculous tangents and hypothetical arguments. I used to be able to tell a good story. Now I just tag along silently.

I am quiet. Quiet is weird. For the first time in my life I actually have something of substance to say, but my mouth is shut. I try to follow their conversations. But eventually I tune out. It's like I am Bella from *Twilight* when Edward ran away and she just sat at the table in the cafeteria for months as everyone else talked around her. My life has become a movie. I feel more like an actress everyday. I am just waiting for the plot twist.

Where will my story go next? It seems to have plateaued at the climax. The real world has returned to normal. But I have been abducted by aliens. I try to learn about civil procedure with the rest of my classmates. They discuss the rules of the litigation game. They play out scenarios to remember who can sue and in which court. They go over the rules of trials and discuss the differences between the Australian, English, American and Canadian legal systems. They argue about which legal TV Shows produce the most accurate depiction of real legal practices. They plan road trips to the Supreme Court. I just sit there staring at my blank page until I find the urge to get up and move.

I always find myself wandering around the Law library. I end up outside with the smokers. None of my friends smoke. But you end up making friends with the regular puffers on campus. It's a nice break. I enjoy the mix of fresh and toxic air. It gives me something to do for five minutes. Then I return -- via the longest route possible -- back to the study chairs. No one else has moved. I pick up my textbook and flick through it. I grab my papers and shuffle them around. I sigh and flick them to the side. Then I tap my pen against the notepad until someone asks me to stop. I then try to draw something to keep my hands busy. I find myself starting to talk about the most bizzare shit but I can't stop. It's like projectile vomit coming out of my mouth. I can tell the crowd isn't engaged, but I just keep going. The librarian comes over to *shhh* me.

I want to make people laugh. I am a pretty good comedian at the moment. But I am just too loud, too vibrant and too frantic to sit in a library. Eventually I pack up my stuff and leave. I find another crowd. I go back to my room and draw another fucking picture. I can't complain. It soothes me. But it isn't solving any of my problems. I have an assessment due tomorrow on tortious liability. I haven't even started it yet. I hate myself for putting it off for so long. I don't know what I am going to do. I guess I could pull an all-nighter and skip the fancy dress party tonight. Or I could just go out, get drunk and tear up the dance floor in my tuxedo or rainbow morphsuit. I like option B.

Manic Barbie

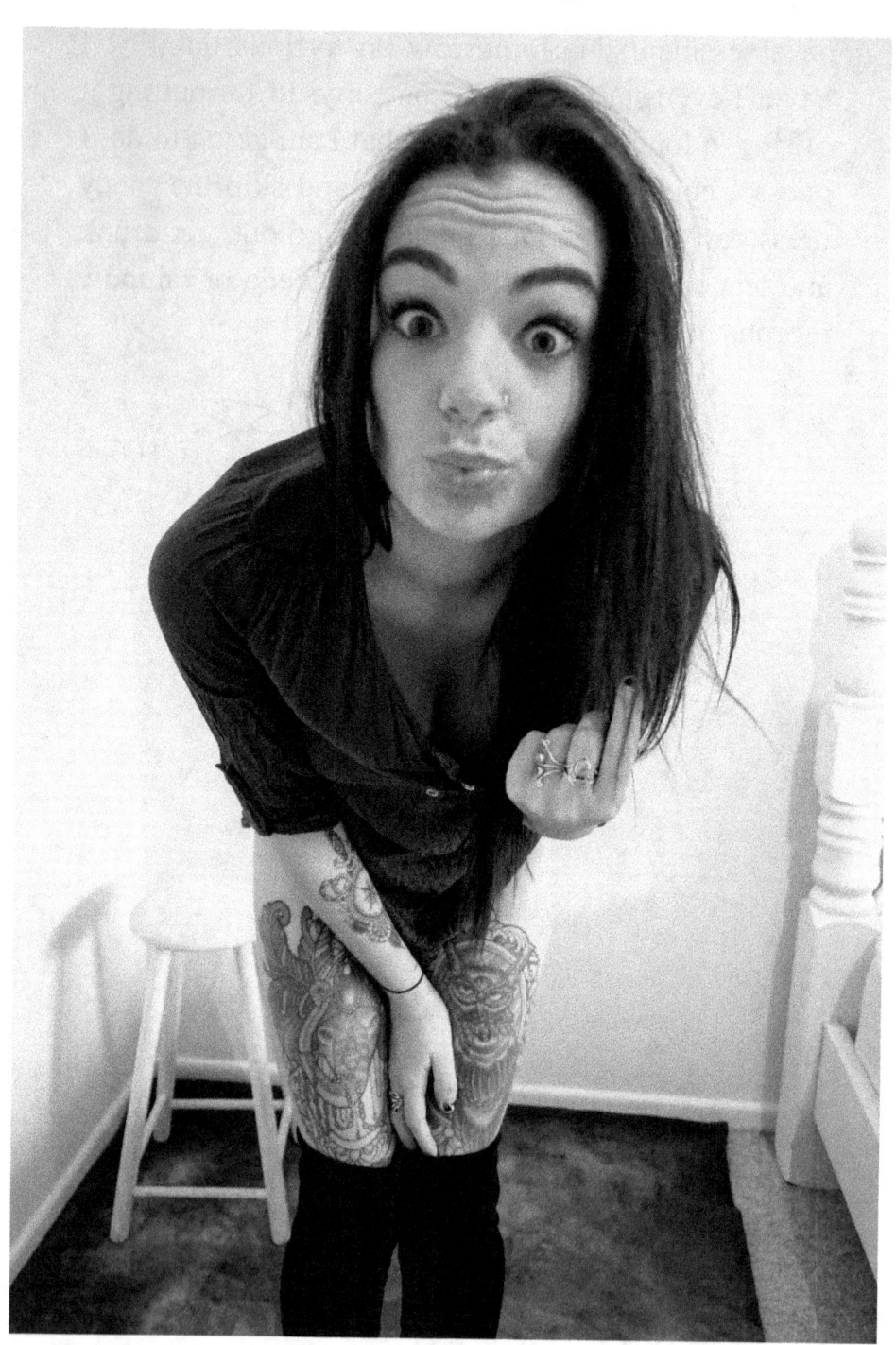

Dear Diary,

Somehow I got my tequila soaked self together and wrote the essay. I honestly don't know how I did it. I spent all morning writing my little ass off. I was hung over to the max! *Ugh.* I felt like shit. It was room cleaning day and the cleaners came in, but my room was a mess. I told them to skip this week. I really wish I hadn't. The smell of vomit still hasn't left my carpet yet. But they can't clean with all this mess. The mountain of clothes on my floor just seems to grow. My wardrobe is nothing more than a place for me to curl up in the dark and hide. I have no idea why I do that. It's like a bird making a nest from discarded robes.

I had put fairy lights across my ceiling and decorated my room. It was like the best house on the street at Christmas time. It is the most envied room on campus. My room is my creative little sanctuary. But now it has just turned into a rubbish dump. I am pretty sure I have been living in this filth long enough. I just can't be fucked dealing with it right now.

I honestly can't believe I got that assignment in. I am relieved to be honest. But also so angry with myself. Why did I do this? Or should I say, why did I do this *again*? What is wrong with me? Why have my priorities changed? Why can't I just get this shit done like everyone else? UGH!!!!!!!

I have taken my sleeping pills and I will soon be off. Night night. I know you're not supposed to drink while taking them … but hey, I don't really care at this point. What is the worst that could happen? I die? It's not really a big deal to me anymore. Death seems inevitable. It is just a matter of time. I am resolved to the fact that the next knock at my door will be the grim reaper.

Hungover Barbie

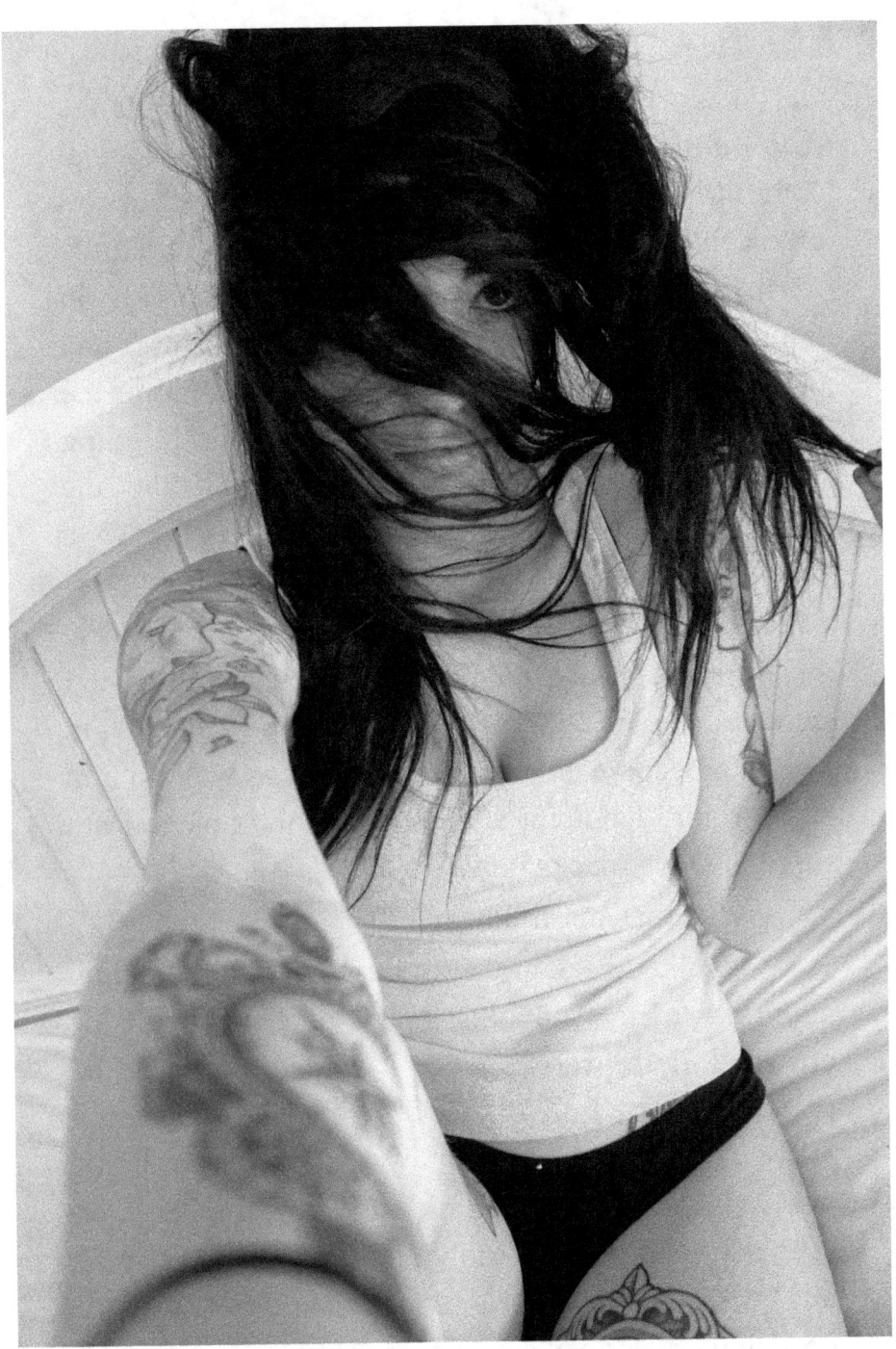

Dear Diary,

I am relieved to have finished classes for the day. I am also relieved to not have any more social commitments. I am done finding excuses to get drunk in crowds. Now I just have a bottle of tequila on my desk. I am however out of the putrid gold liquid. I walked to the local corner store and purchased a bottle of white tequila. The smell of the yellow stuff just makes me want to barf. I am going to have to start going to different stores. I think the clerk at this one is beginning to notice I have a serious problem.

I paid for my booze and walked into the supermarket next door. I am prepared today. I purchased a bag of lemons, limes and salt. If I'm going to become an alcoholic, I might as well do it in style, right? I bought another pack of smokes. I am on to the forty packs now.

What has my life become?

I walked back to uni and tried to avoid drawing attention to my shopping as I walked through the crowded dorm room halls. I smiled politely and pretended to be fine. In fact I pretended to be *great*. I joked and interacted with my friends like nothing was wrong. I have started hiding everything, anxious to evade the people I know and extinguish all small talk. All I ever want is to get into my room, close the door and crack open a bottle.

I am grateful for my shot glass. It makes it easier to numb the pain. I take one, two, three and four before I can even breathe. I gulp some juice just to get the taste out of my mouth and then I down another few. I pop some pain killers too. I like the way they thin my blood and get me drunk a lot quicker and off of a lot less. It makes the whole process a lot more economical. My stomach is starting to become putrid from the excess of alcohol I consume daily.

What to do next? All I can think of is wallowing in my own self-pity. I should be studying. I am in law school after all. But my grades are terrible, my attendance is poor and I can't study because I spend all night awake with my terrible thoughts.

Drinking every day started out innocent enough. It started out as a way to cope with Jo's death, but now it's just become a habit. It's been months since she passed away and I am still not okay. The drinking stopped being about grieving for her death and now it's just an escape from the reality that she is gone and never coming back.

The worst part of this though? It's not even working anymore. All it does is make me think more about how stupid this whole thing is and what will happen if my parents find out.

I stare down at the empty bottle of vodka and

wipe my tears away. I am alone in my dorm room, drinking way too much to try and cope with this semester. Jo's passing has really shaken me up. I can't seem to keep myself together anymore, I'm losing hope that any good will come out of this year. It's not fair what happened to her. But it happened and there is nothing that can be done about it.

I watch another tear fall on my sheets and then take another shot to stop the thoughts racing through my head like an express train with no breaks. *I am too far gone;* I think to myself as I look at the bottle of tequila in my hand. I take another shot. I look around to see if anyone has noticed. There is no one here but me and my regrets.

The walls are closing in on me and every day feels different than the last. I am beginning to hate myself with a passion. I despise this train wreck I have become. I am disappointed in myself. I just gazed across the room and l caught a glimpse of my reflection in the mirror. I felt a barrage of emotions: shame, anger, self-hatred. All because I can't keep up with this downward spiral anymore.

I collapse into bed and bury my head into the pillow. Everything is overwhelming and it is suffocating me to death. And now here I am looking in the mirror with cracks through my foundation that no amount of concealer would help cover up because they are on the inside; mirrors don't lie about such things when we know what we see is not going to change for a while if ever again …

I close my eyes and pull the doona up over my head. I image being submerged under water in a pond. I'm lying on my back staring at the surface I can't seem to touch. I watch the light flicker through the crisp water's edge. It's bright and blinding but mesmerising. I see distorted faces staring down at me through the lily pads. I can see them but they can't see me. They see

I scream "Help!"

"Please, someone help!"

No one hears my pleas. They are too busy admiring the beauty of the surface to care what lays beneath. I wonder how many years I could lay here beneath the surface, beneath the covers before someone notices me. I want someone to dive in and pull me out. I want someone to notice that I am drowning.

I want someone to look beneath the surface and uncover the ugly truth, that beneath all this, there is a struggle. Me.

Self-loathing Barbie

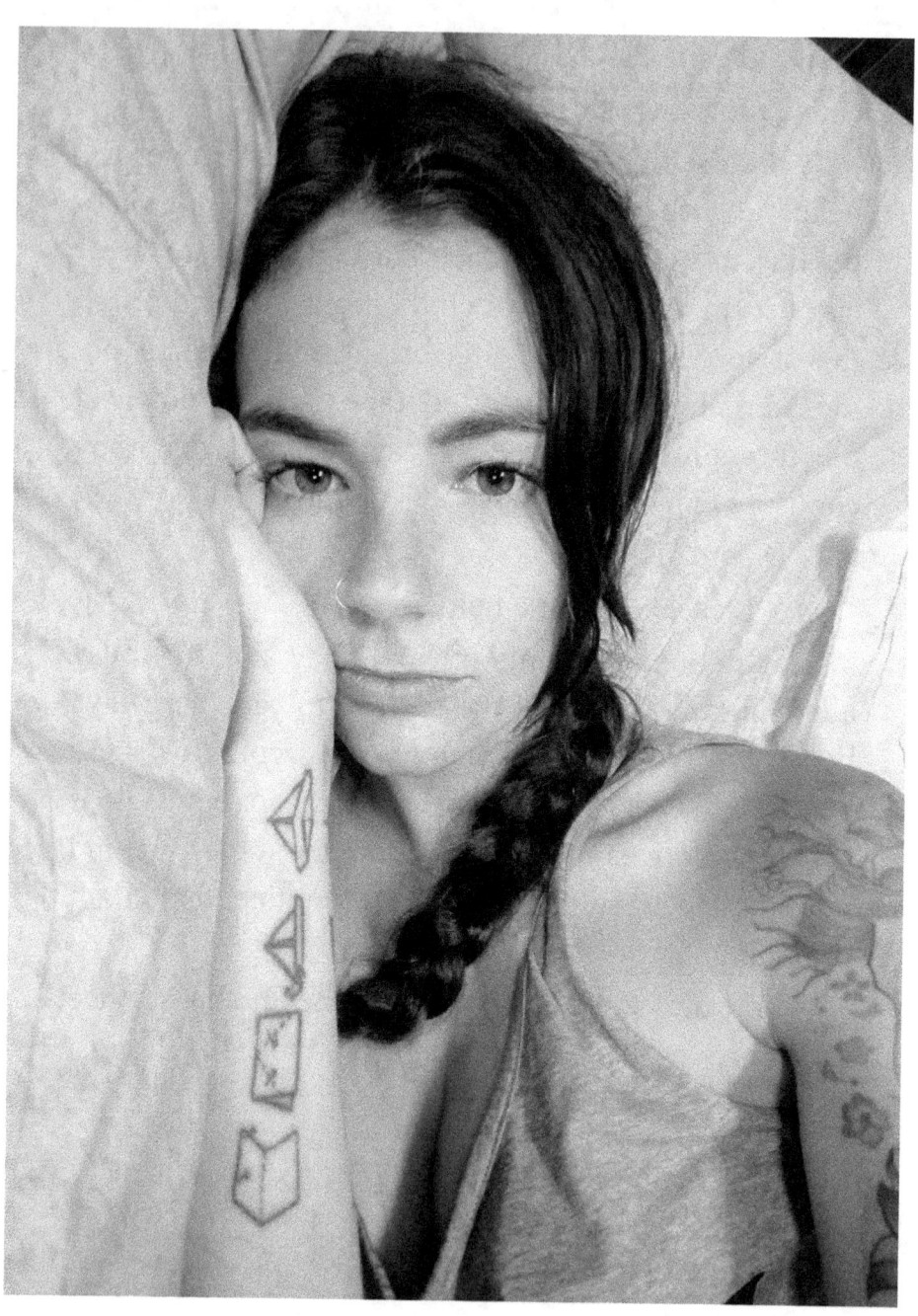

Dear Diary,

I woke up with a killer headache this morning. It's 11am and my tutorial is at 1pm today. My eyes are bloodshot and my head is throbbing from too much alcohol.

The room spun around as soon as I moved my head an inch. As I tried to get out of bed I stumbled over my giant washing pile of clothes on the floor. The clothes were stained in brownish orange spots of vomit smeared all over them. Ugh. Why do I keep doing this to myself?

I groaned aloud before clumsily making my way to the communal bathrooms. I could feel how empty my body had become as the alcohol wore off and all that was left for me to do was think about what happened, over and over again. I got into the shower to wash away any evidence that may have suggested how much I drank last night. Turns out I'd vomited all over myself in my sleep ...

The hot water soothed my skin and helped clear out some of the fog in my brain. The only downside to the fog lifting is that with it I began to feel again. My safety blanket of numbness was ripped off like a Band-Aid and I was once again an open wound.

I collapsed on the shower floor and cried. I curled up in the foetal position on the cold tiles and tried to imagine the water washing away all my pain. But no matter how hard I tried; it was like I could never get clean. My body felt heavy and tired, like a boulder had been placed on top of my shoulders. It's too much to carry and life seems so pointless because with each day the weight just gets heavier and heavier until finally I won't be able to take it anymore

After what seemed like an eternity, I got out of the shower and dressed myself for class. I tried to brush off as much eye makeup smeared on my face as possible before heading out the door for my morning cigarette. Just as habitual as the thoughts of death that cross my mind. Who knew there were an endless amount of scenarios you could come up with when planning your own demise?

I closed my eyes. I imagined that I was standing at the edge of a cliff. The sun shone through my hair and I felt the wind on my skin for just one last time before I started to fall. I fell and closed my eyes waiting to hit the ground. But I didn't. I opened my eyes to check. I was still there. The ground was firmly beneath my feet and I was unfortunately still alive and in agony.

Hungover Barbie

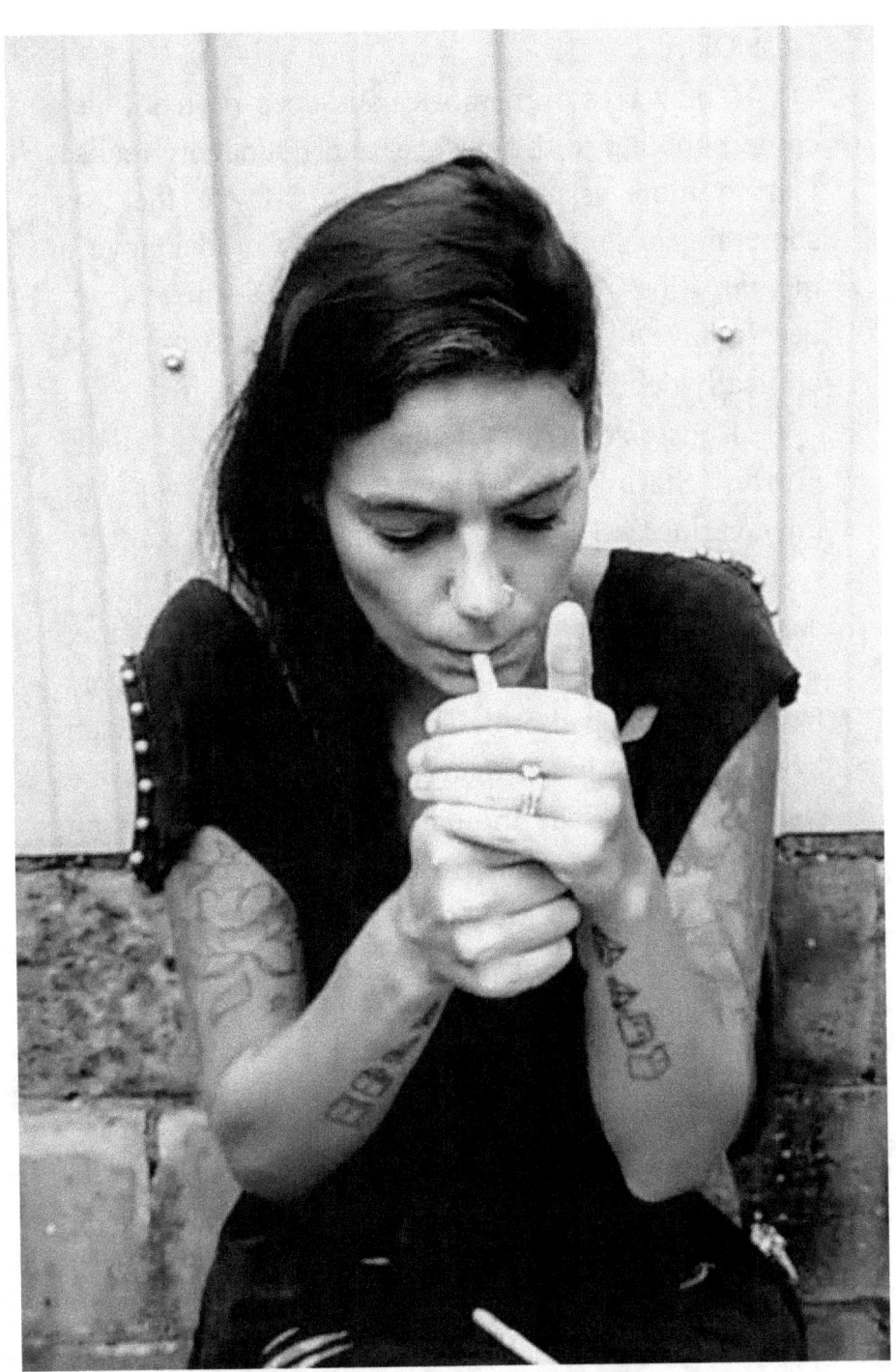

Dear Diary,

The waves of memories and deep-rooted issues come bubbling to the surface, and I suddenly realise I have more issues than vogue. Maybe there is something else going on with me? Could I have a mental illness? The thought terrifies me. Never before have I ever contemplated the fact I might be clinically depressed.

I just stood in my bathroom, staring at the mirror. Staring into my eyes. My gaze was unwavering as I tried to see something that can't be seen. But there should be something, right? There has to be a mental illness lurking inside me, somewhere deep down, like one of those monsters from under the bed or behind the closet door; hidden from sight but always ready to grab me when no one else is looking. The thought terrifies me more than anything I've ever imagined before. What if they can't find it? What if they don't believe me?

I couldn't get up and start my day because I was dreading what new idea would hit me today. It's like every single time I tried to think about anything it turned into an issue that had to be dealt with. My thoughts are being pulled in so many different directions today, but there is one thought that keeps coming back – *am I insane?*

The face of mental illness, one title I never thought I'd have. Once upon a time a Miss Universe beauty queen, now crowned Miss Insanity! *crowd cheers*. Note to self: buy a crown, I think I deserve one. It would look good with my too-depressed-to-brush-my-hair outfit, and I can rock it when I binge-watch TV in bed for days.

My mind is playing mean tricks on me, and I seem to be at the mercy of something else ... But what? I don't know ... Something is controlling me from someplace deep within. It is wrapped around my core pulling tighter with each breath I take. I feel like the baby I wish I was, with the umbilical cord wrapped around my neck.

This heavy feeling in my chest is constricting my lungs. I can't breathe. What is happening to me? I want to cry all the time. But instead I lay on the floor of my uni dorm room silently screaming for help.

Today I spent hours from the time I left the afternoon lecture on property law 'til what is now almost 12am on top of a pile of clothes on the floor. Whether they are dirty or not, I have no idea. My senses are dulled. Or perhaps the smell of dirty washing is simply snuffed out by last week's vomit rotting on the carpet. I don't know if the smell will ever leave. It's just a reminder of the mess I have become and the end of my relationship with vodka Double Black cans.

I didn't think about much during those hours

when I was collapsed on the floor. Time just seemed to fly by, although I barely noticed. I blinked and four hours had passed. My eyes were open, but I saw nothing. I was afraid to close them for fear of what I might see. Besides, it took far too much effort to keep them shut. I didn't have the energy my face muscles demanded to execute that action. I was aware of how heavy my body felt. My head was the heaviest of all. Yet somehow I also felt like I was floating. Just bobbing about like Terry Jo Duperrault in the middle of the ocean, lost at sea.

I am tormented day and night by this dark overbearing presence. I can't run from my demons. They have moved into my mind and simply refuse to leave. They are squatters that have become the most annoying housemates I've ever had! And I've had a lot of batshit crazy housemates! I can't hide from them either. I am trapped in my own body. I couldn't escape this ... this ... whatever this is ... *I don't know!*

When will my world be normal again?

Miss Mentally Ill Barbie

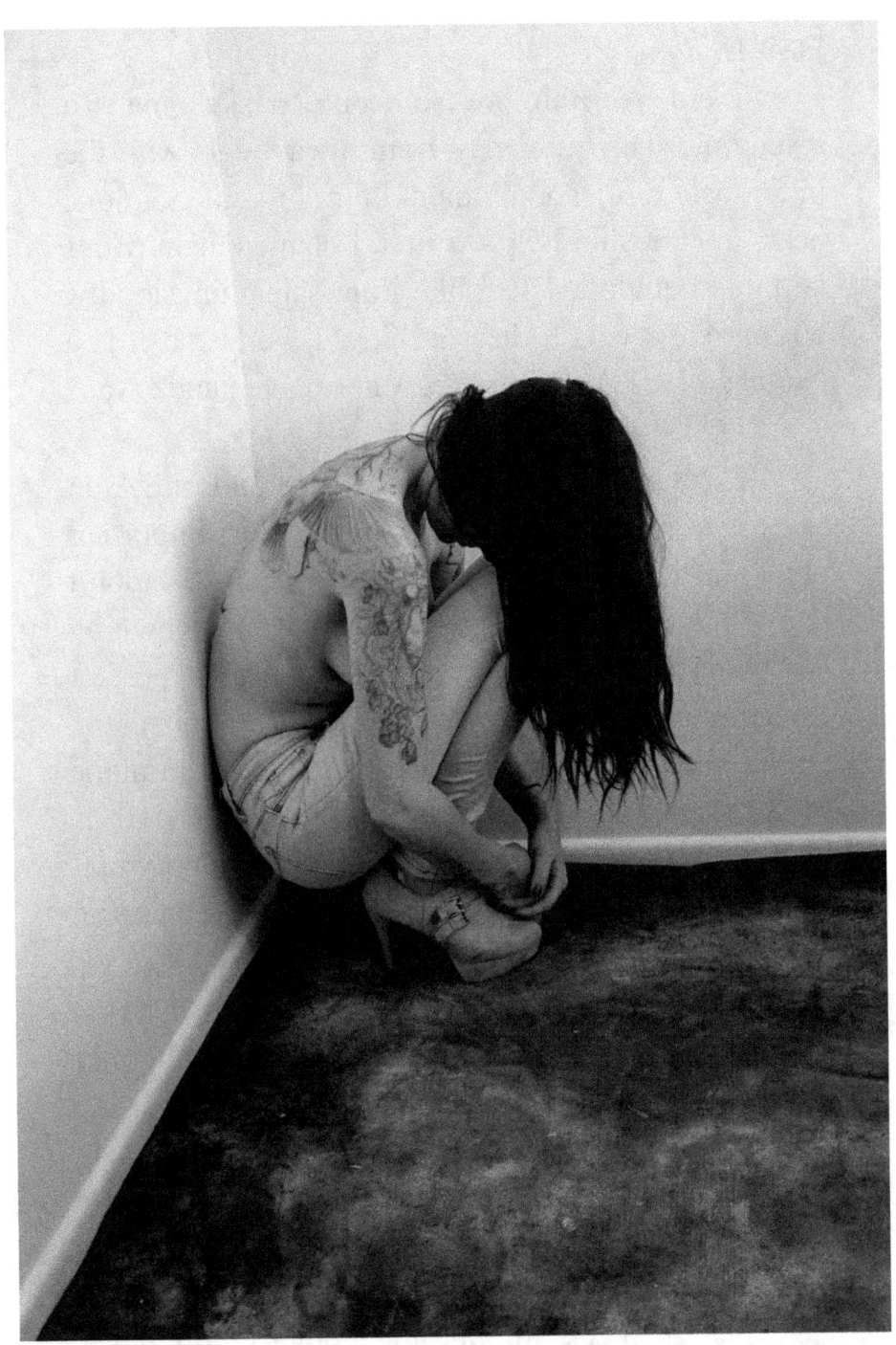

Dear Diary,

I am yearning for someone to save me. To rescue me. Day after day I am always left with the bitter taste of disappointment on my tongue. No one hears my cries for help. At first, I blamed them. But I know I shouldn't. I feel like I am screaming loudly, but no one seems to hear a thing. I wonder if it is a language barrier. Do they just not understand? Am I speaking Chinese?

I use every descriptive sentence under the sun to explain my despair, except for the most important phrase of all, "I need help". But for what? I don't know. Something is wrong with me. I am drowning and then soaring, and I watch the walls of my perfect life crumble around me. I lay atop my pile of rubble and destruction, head in hands and I cry. I am alone in this war. I know I need a hero. That is obvious. I want my dad to save me. After all, he's the only real hero I've ever known. But when I need him most he is nowhere to be found.

I called my dad today to tell him for the first time that I wasn't okay. It was short, but certainly not sweet. He has always been a man of few words. I am not. People always told me I would be able to talk underwater with marbles in my mouth. Most people listened to me when I talked, but my father was a hard nut to crack. Dad tries, I guess, in his own way. He calls to check in, but the conversation never really lasts more than a few minutes. It is like he does his civic duty to make sure I am okay and that is about the extent of his conversational comfort zone. I try to push him beyond that, but he normally ends the conversation saying he has to go back to work. Our conversations lately have been getting shorter and shorter.

We used to be close. But now we are strangers to one another. We live in separate worlds. He isn't really interested in the social life of a female uni student, and as his daughter, I'm not exactly going to tell him the details of it either. I am at law school, and he is a mechanic. The concepts I am learning in class are a little difficult for him to grasp. I am not saying he is stupid. Because he is not. I don't think anyone would understand the legal system unless you studied it well. Even then it is an enigma.

We always speak about news and current events, but never about us. I guess it is too uncomfortable for him. It is clear he doesn't want to hear what I have to say and his life really does not interest me that much either.

I desperately wanted to tell him that I'm really not okay. But he just brushed it off telling me I would be alright. "Just give it time," he encouraged.

The fact of the matter is, I'm not alright and I haven't been for a long time. I think he just thinks because he has only heard about it recently, it has just happened. But it has been going on for months. When he directly asked me if I was okay, I replied "no". He then proceeded to ask me why and I told him I didn't know. I found it hard to explain exactly what was going on in my life. How do you tell your father you want to die?

He quickly ended the call after that. I was left sitting on my dorm room floor. I still had my phone in my hand. I didn't know what to do. So I cried. I felt my stomach churning. I couldn't breathe. I just cried. Not in a pretty actress kind of way. I cried like a wailing mother who'd just watched her child die.

I understand it probably made him feel uncomfortable, perhaps even worried sick. But avoiding me wasn't really helping. Regardless of what he really felt, it portrayed a message that he didn't care.

I have never felt so unloved. I just want to scream "Stop asking me to trust you while I'm coughing up water from the last time you let me drown!"

I have no faith that he will save me. He just doesn't know what he is talking about.

Desperate Daughter Barbie

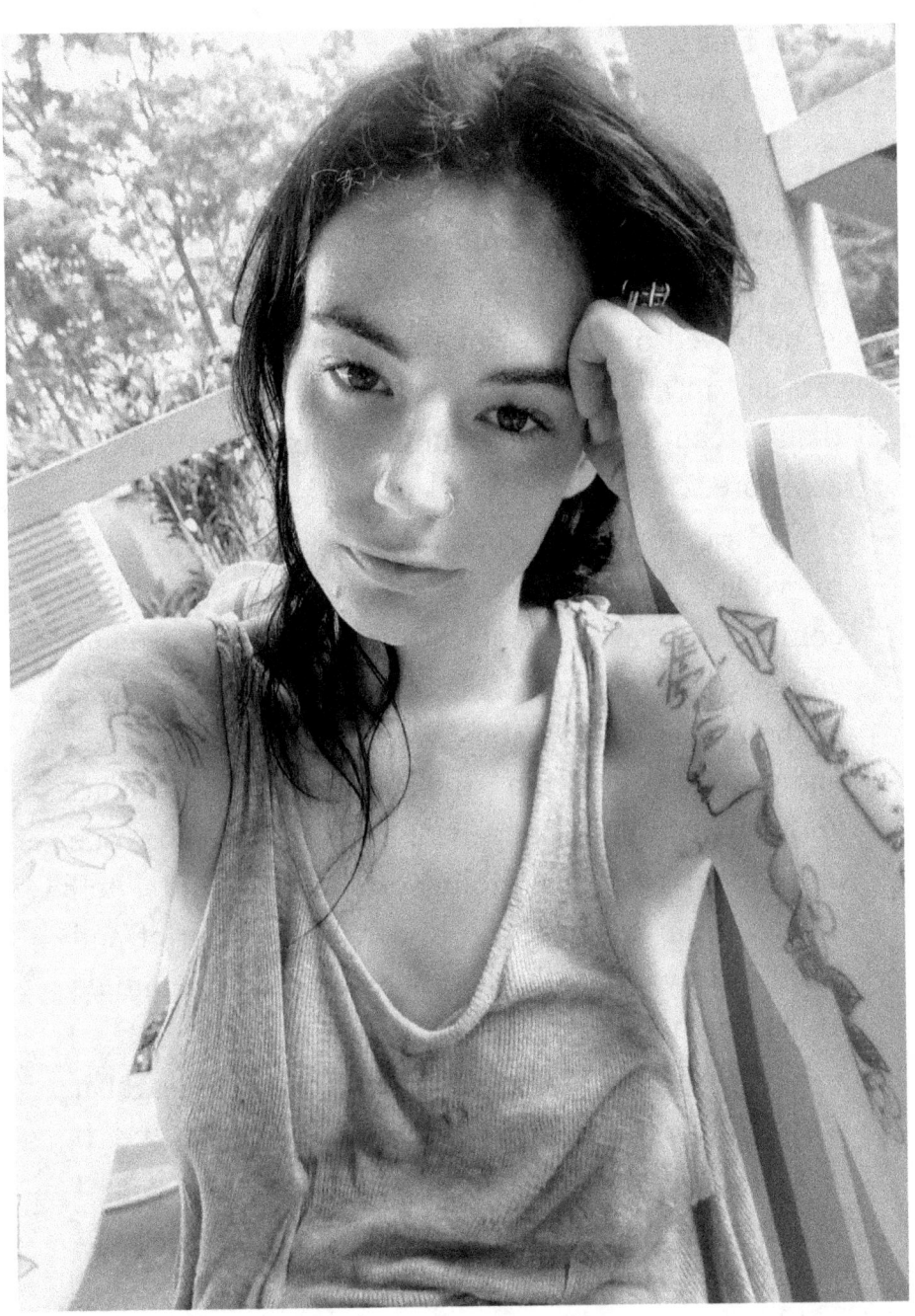

Dear Diary,

I feel numb and empty as I move through the days. The grey time between morning and evening seems to go on forever. The place where my life doesn't really exist anymore, to me or anyone else.

My body is a mere shell of what it used to be. A hollowed out home for the thoughts that haunted me day in and day out. The pain is so much more than I can ever endure until I just can't take it anymore…

I ran to the bathroom in tears. I still had a can of vodka mix in my hand. My friends tried to comfort me as I burst through the corridor and collapsed on the floor. Their concern and willingness to help was honourable. But they couldn't even understand why I felt so bad because they didn't know what had happened. How could anyone understand what was going on? What could I tell them? "I am drowning in my own sea of grief and guilt"? How could they comprehend the magnitude of my downfall?

The water is so much deeper than I thought it was. It's like there is no bottom to this sea, no end. It just goes on and on, pulling me down with it as I struggle to get back up through the waves of hopelessness that slam against me as they rise higher and higher until they are all around me – drowning every last sliver of light from my eyes, blinding me in darkness.

    I can feel the water pressing against my body, crushing me into a ball. I had thought that this time would be different, but it's not. It is just another one of those days where there is nothing to live for and everything to die from. The waves are too strong and at some point they have swallowed me whole.

    It feels like the entire world is crashing down; all the pain I've ever felt in my life is coming back as quick flashes of memories that haunt me in every waking moment of my day-to-day routine. Every second feels like an eternity before I finally let go …

Depressed Barbie

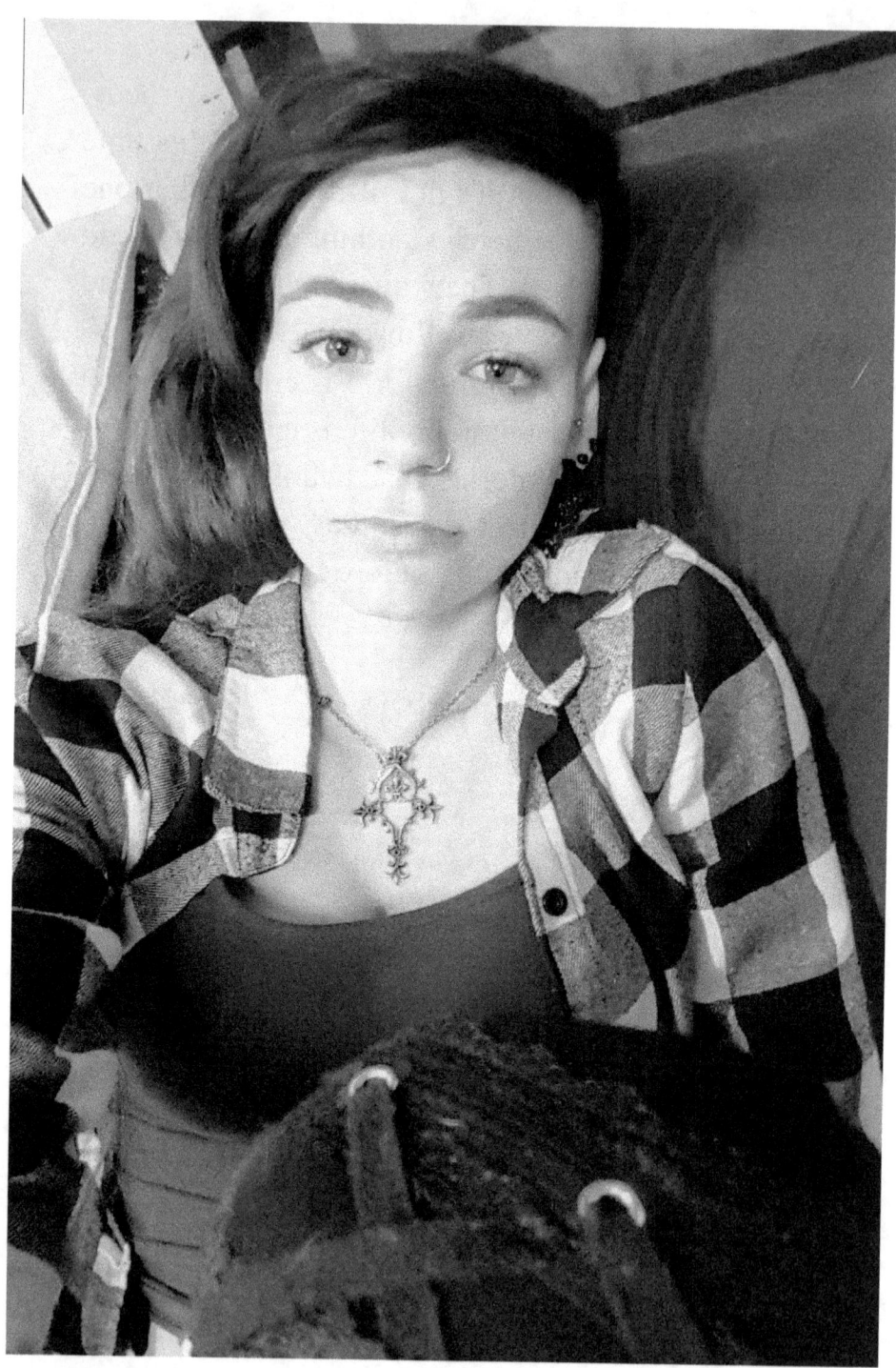

Dear Diary,

A friend of a friend confronted me today. She scolded me for making the rest of our friendship group worry. I was told that one of my closest friends was extremely worried about me. Apparently she had been waking through the night and sneaking into my dorm room just to make sure I was alright.

I was shocked. I had no idea anyone cared that much. I had no idea anyone even knew how bad things had gotten. But then again I wasn't trying to hide it. I was only surprised because not one person had said anything until now. It had been months! I was almost half a year into my downward spiral.

This concerned phone call came from the person I least liked in my friendship group. But I did have a newfound respect for her. I knew why she was the one to break the dam. She was not afraid of confrontation. That made me understand how scared they all were of my reaction.

I realised I was being selfish. We've already had one friend not wake up this semester. It was rather devastating to realise you will never see someone again, someone you had just seen the day before. You never really think about that when it's you about to drop. I'm not suicidal. I'm not actively trying to take my life; I just don't care whether I live or die.

If I am being completely honest though, I am a ticking time bomb. I hadn't realised I wasn't hiding it as well as I thought until now. I have been open about how much I am struggling. But as the 'appropriate' mourning period after my mother's death has run out, so has the empathy others have for me. Am I expected to just get over it? How long is the appropriate time to mourn? It seems a month or perhaps two for a close family member is the time frame you have to grieve. After that you are expected to just magically move on with your life. I can't.

I think it's about time I take her advice and do something more about this. I need to go to the doctor. Where else can I turn?

Wake Up Call Barbie

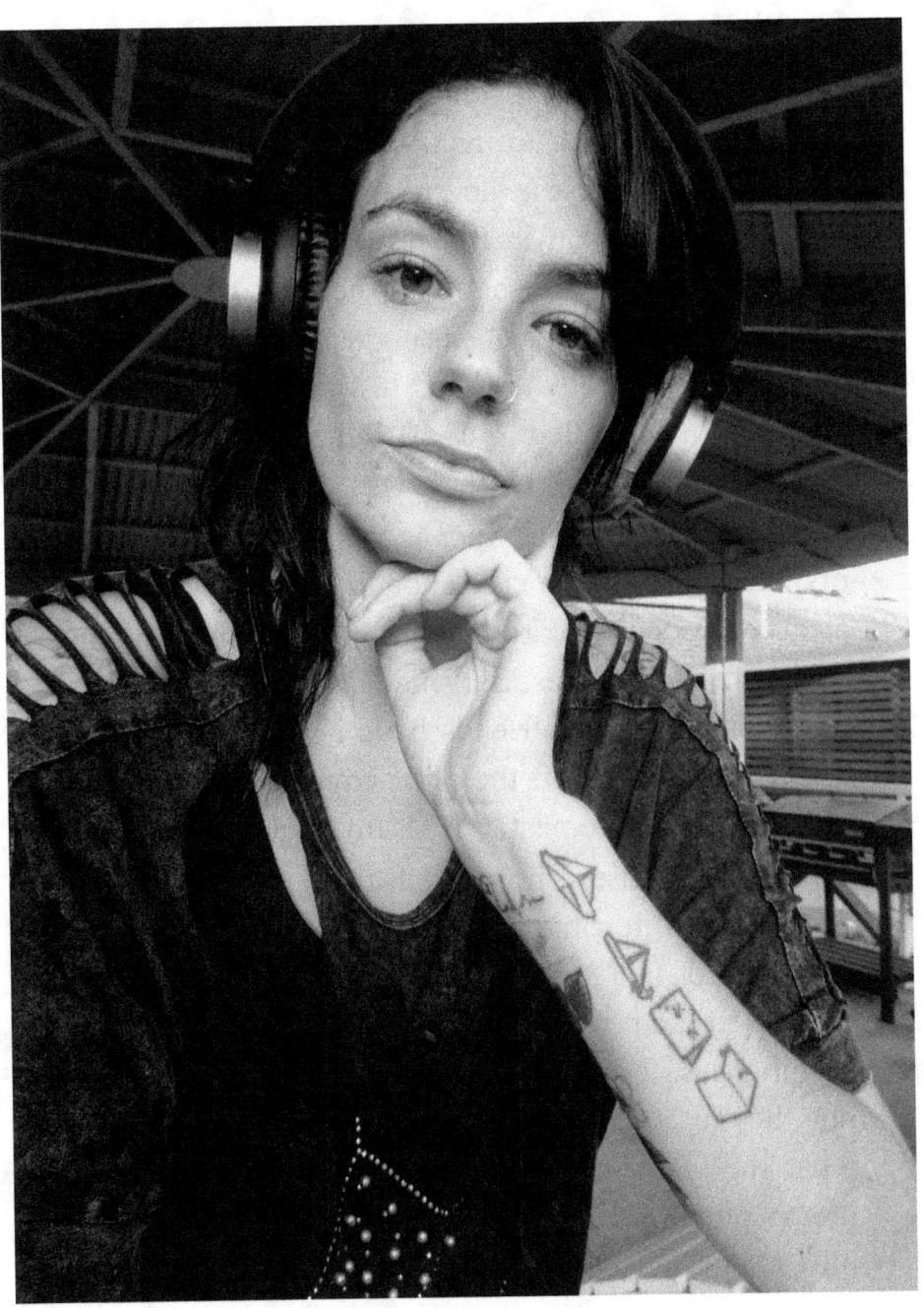

Dear Diary,

After being confronted last night I texted my friend this morning to thank her for being there for me. Even though she doesn't know anything about what was going on in my head. She responded by telling me that we all have our demons to deal with sometimes, and part of caring is doing something about them if you need to. It was a wakeup call. Literally; she called me at 2am. Oh who am I kidding, I wasn't sleeping anyway.

The last thing I want is for this to be hurting my friends. If I don't care enough about myself, then at the very least I care enough about them to make some drastic changes. Self-medicating my pain isn't going to cut it. My friends have held my hair back and picked me up off the floor covered in vomit too many times this semester. It has to stop.

I can't believe how much this is impacting my friends. I feel terrible for putting them through all of this. It's not fair that they have to help me take care of myself and watch as I slowly fade away into nothingness. They deserve so much better than me, but they're stuck with someone who doesn't know what she wants or needs anymore. It is not fair for me to put them through this. I might deserve this misery but they certainly do not.

It's time to make a change before it's too late. I am going to do something about it. I'm in a dire place. I don't know what to do, but there is one thing that seems clear – I can't go on like this. There still may be time for me to make it out of the darkness and into the light.

I am going to reach out to the university medical clinic. I don't know who else to call.

Terrible Friend Barbie

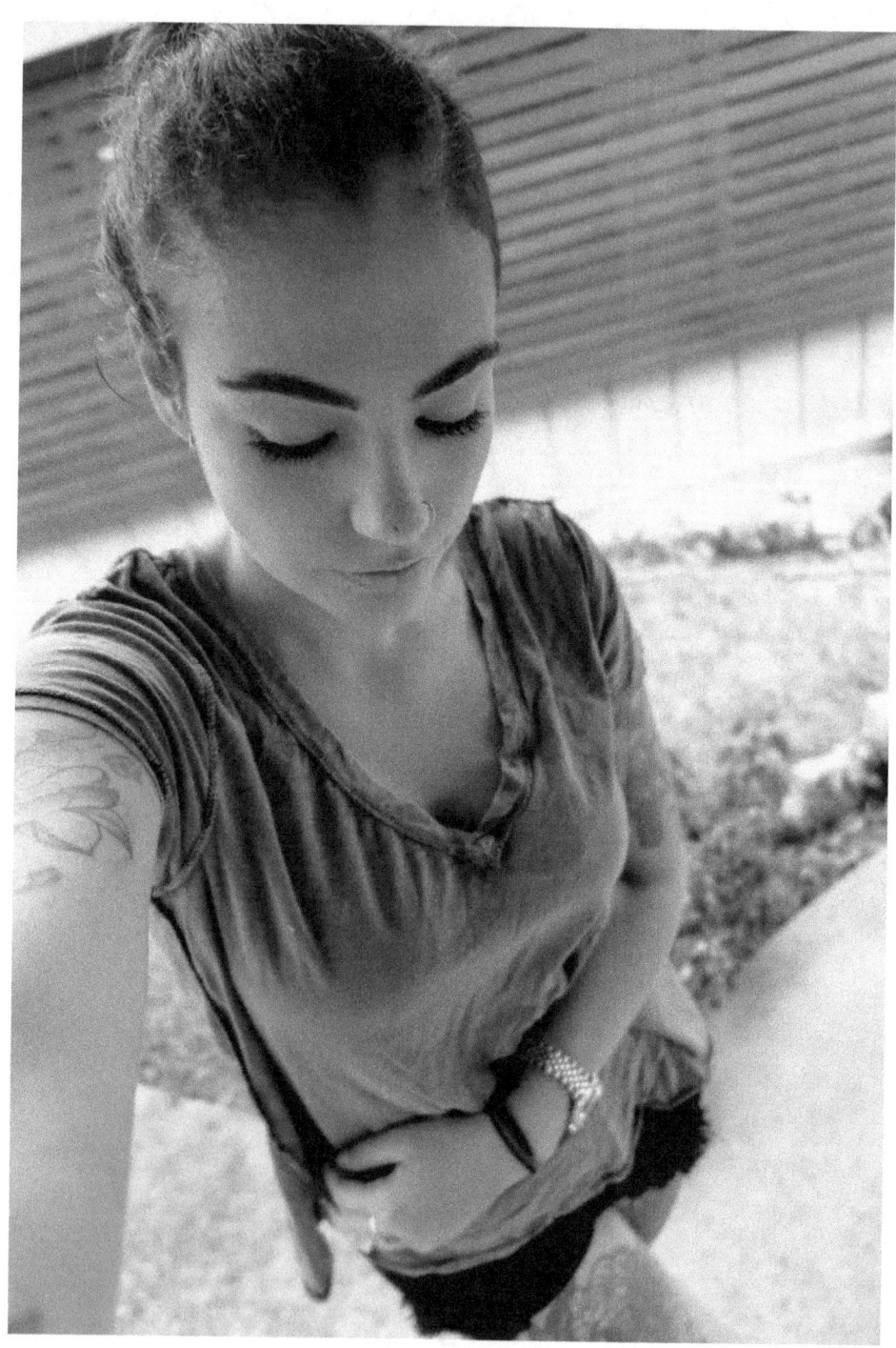

Dear Diary,

I left my dorm room this morning and embarked on the greatest journey of my life. I was nervous and excited. I walked across campus to the university medical centre. I told the receptionist that I had arrived then took a seat in the waiting room. I was filled with anxious anticipation. I had no idea what to expect. I didn't even really know what I was going to say. I had prepared the conversation with my doctor over and over again in my head. I'd rehearsed the dialogue like an actor preparing for a play. But this was no act. Not even a Shakespearean tragedy. This was the most real I had been in a long time.

I waited for forty-five minutes and tried to remain invisible. But since this was the uni medical centre and I knew nearly everyone on campus, I was singled out by many acquaintances. The chair next to me was like a revolving hot seat. I felt like a talk show host interviewing my next guest. I found it hard to put up my façade that I had tried all morning to let down for this appointment. I had let the wall come down and it was now just a thin veil I was sure was invisible. When they finally called my name I looked up with surprise. The familiar face of my uni GP greeted me with a smile. I tried to return one but I am still not quite sure if it ever manifested on my face. My last guest yelled across the room 'Good

Luck!' as I departed the waiting area. I turned to acknowledge the gesture, but luckily turned the corner before they could catch a glimpse of my concerned look.

As I walked into the office my doctor motioned for me to sit in the patient's chair. He closed the door behind him and walked around me to sit behind his desk. I sat in the chair across from my doctor and he stared at me a minute before breaking the ice.

"What can I do for you today?"

The only words I could mutter were, "'m not okay".

That was when I realised the hardest bit was yet to come. Those four words I had been dreading to speak for months were only the beginning. His response was where the real challenge began. "Well, what's going on?" He enquired.

The floor shook beneath my feet. I could hear the air being exhaled out of my nostrils. I could feel my heart beating rapidly in my chest. I was nervous and a little scared. Why was he looking at me like that? He had been sitting there for a while now, waiting for me to speak up. but the more time passed, the more uncomfortable I felt. I tried to respond but it seemed as though the words were stuck in my mouth. It was as if the air had been sucked out of the room. I stared at him blankly. I had no response.

What was wrong with me? A question I had pondered for months. The exact question he was supposed to answer! I had planned this day for weeks. I woke up at the crack of dawn to get ready so that I would be completely fresh and rehearsed. I had repeated those words "I am not okay" over a hundred times just so that I knew I could speak them on cue. I wasn't prepared for this. I hadn't expected anything to come next.

I stared at him blankly and he waited for me to speak. But what should I say? How can you explain how it feels when you've felt this way for months on end, as if everything that had ever made sense to you suddenly didn't anymore?

"I – uh –" My voice cracked, as if it physically couldn't make any sound. "I don't know." I whispered under my breath. It was barely audible, but I knew he heard it because his eyes softened and then he leaned forward with compassion.

"That's okay. We can figure it out together." he assured me.

I nodded and took a deep calming breath. I felt the tears welling in my eyes begin to subside. I felt relief for the first time since this all began. I felt like things would finally be okay again.

I felt like I had been given a lifeline. Provided

with a float and a chance to catch my breath with the promise of rescue. I had hope. For the first time in months I didn't feel alone.

I felt as if the clouds had parted and the sky was blue again. I could see a way out, even if I didn't know what it was. I had a plan. I had actionable steps that I could take to regain control of my life.

Reaching out Barbie

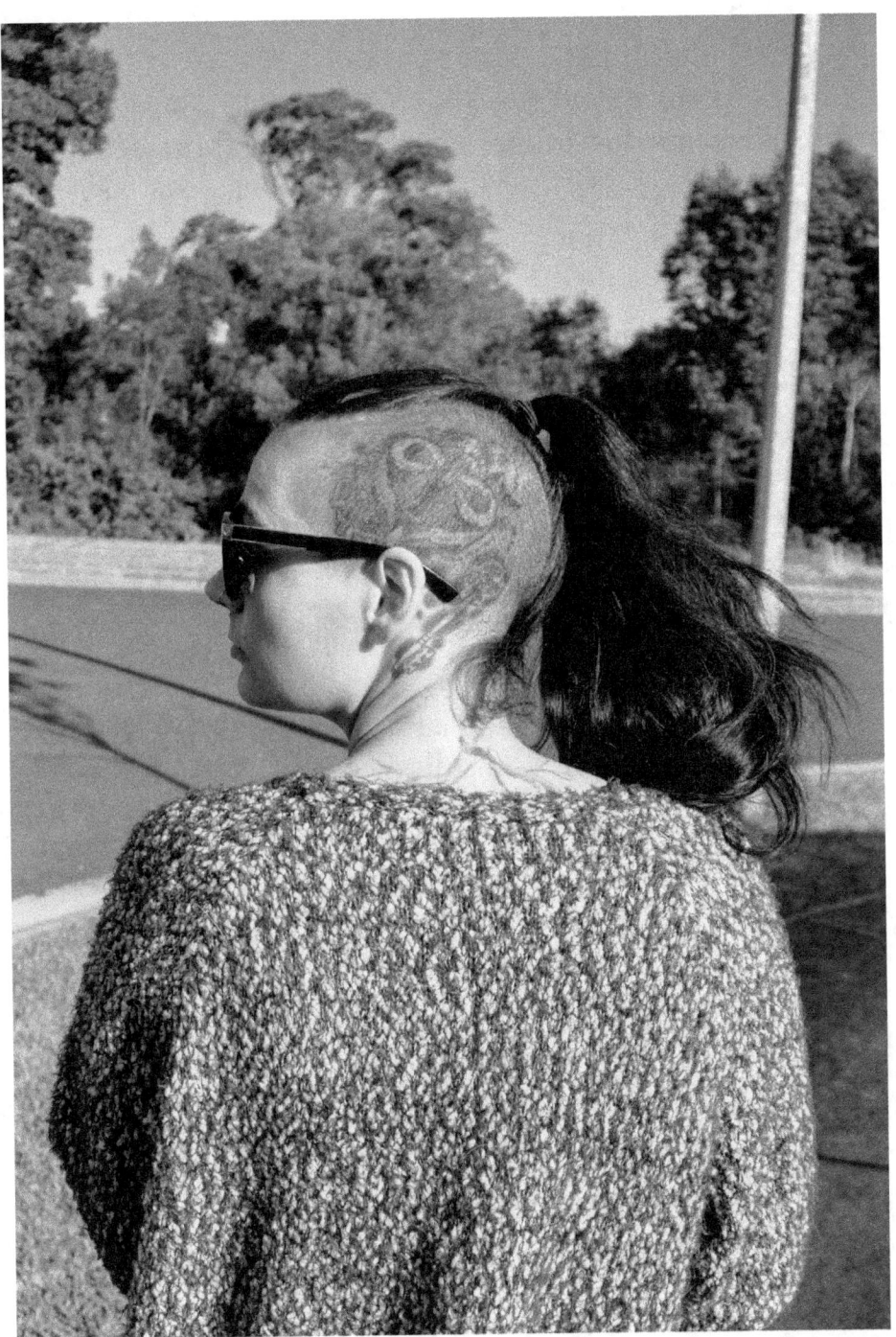

Dear Diary,

Today I had my first ever therapy session. I walked into the office of my new therapist feeling apprehensive about what was going to happen next. In the waiting room I sat feeling more nervous by the minute.

A side door opened to a consultation room and my new therapist called my name. I got up and slowly walked up to the door in front of me and took a deep breath before entering. He introduced himself and waved for me to have a seat. The man sitting across from me explained how therapy works and offered me an opportunity to get started on my own journey towards recovery.

"Hi, so why did you come today?" he asked in a tone that would be dismissive if it wasn't for his gentle smile and warm brown eyes.

I shifted in my seat uncomfortably, trying to find the perfect words. He gazed at me with eager anticipation. I didn't know where to start. I had a hard time deciding what was important information to share. What facts really mattered? There didn't seem to be anything real or tangible to begin with. Except Jo's passing of course. So I started there.

We discussed her death and my movements since. He listened as he wrote notes in the journal on his lap. It wasn't long before he wanted to start discussing my childhood. So I gave him my origin story.

I was born in the suburbs of Sydney with my Mum, Dad and little sister, but on my ninth birthday we moved to a quiet little town on the Northern Beaches. We had a five acre property that I absolutely loved. I was such an outdoors, animal and nature loving kid. My chores consisted of feeding the chickens, collecting eggs and cleaning their nests.

Not too long after I got my first horse. I did competitive horse riding for years. I rode motorbikes too. A hobby my father preferred I pursue. "I prefer a horse you can turn off", he always said. "It's less dangerous." I know most people wouldn't think motocross is safe but if you compare it to the number of times I fell off my horses … then chances are I would have received less broken ribs and concussions.

My therapist then wanted to know more about my relationships with my family. I told him I had a great time with my parents growing up, especially with my dad. We would do all sorts of things together like fishing and fixing things around the house. Although I didn't have the best relationship with my mother. She always seemed emotionally distant and I never felt like she liked me very much. Especially after my grandmother died. Something seemed to break in her. She had violent mood swings and would turn into a monster. A dragon with a fiery tongue spitting hurtful insults. The phrases "Go kill yourself you fucking cunt I wish you were dead!" and "I hate you; I wish you were never born!" come to mind.

I am sure at one point they hurt me. But after a while you get used to it. I watched disbelief come across my therapist's face as I shrugged it off.

"Surely that would have been traumatic for you?" he asked.

"I guess so," I responded. We all learnt to just kind of laugh it off like she was a joke. I couldn't take her seriously. She was a short stocky woman. Far shorter than me by the time I reached my teenage years. She didn't really project an image of someone to be feared. It was kind of pathetic really.

"Right." My therapist nodded. Moving on, he asked me about my dad.

I told him he was my hero, until I went on a student exchange at sixteen to Germany. After the twelve month program I returned, a different, more mature person. I was nearly an adult by then. I had less tolerance for mum's bullshit. So I stood up for myself and faced confrontation head on. I feel like he resented me for leaving him to deal with her. I had been the centre of her frustration and the direction of blame always laid with me. I guess they realised that when I left. Suddenly it was everyone else's fault mum was a psycho.

Things were rough for a while then. I had to finish off my last two years of high school so that I could graduate and get into university. They didn't make it easy for me though. I briefly recounted some key moments of frustration. They kicked me out numerous times because, as dad said, I was unwilling to tow the party line. What that meant I don't know. But it sort of boiled down to: I'd either put up with the abuse at home, and keep my mouth shut, or I didn't have the right to live with them.

It never really seemed fair to me, so I moved in with my best friend's mum. That's why her passing was so hard for me. She gave me shelter and loved me when my own family couldn't. She treated me like a daughter and embraced me with unconditional love.

It was hard to support myself financially while finishing high school and keeping up my grades. I worked almost full time at a phone shop to survive. I don't exactly know why, but my parents couldn't handle the fact that I was just fine without them. They felt a need to destroy me and demonise me in the eyes of everyone they knew. It was as if their pride wouldn't allow me to succeed without them. They did things like take my car that I bought off me, steal all the money from my bank account and take back every item of clothing I owned including my school clothes. I guess they had a right to since they'd bought most of it, but it was rather inconvenient and another layer of stress I didn't need.

"Sounds like you had it rough," he said. I was stunned. I never thought of it like that. It was what it was, normal to me. "That is not normal," he assured me.

I didn't believe him. I couldn't otherwise my whole life had been a lie.

I don't remember the exact words he used but it was something along the lines of "It's no surprise you are 'fucked up'. You have had a lot to deal with and that type of upbringing can create an immense amount of distress for anyone to process."

"But it all happened so suddenly. Why now and never before?" It didn't make sense.

"Times up," he said. "Let's make an appointment for next week."

I left his office feeling confused. Had I had an abusive childhood? Wasn't it a normal one? I thought it was good. I mean I knew it was painful and hurt, but didn't everyone experience the same?

I looked back at my past and realised there was a lot missing. It felt like there were holes in my memory. Each little video that played in my head was like a slice of Swiss cheese.

I remember being ten collecting the chicken's eggs in my red raincoat and gumboots. Filling my pockets with all the eggs I could find. But that memory began to burn through as I walked into the kitchen and entered a screaming match. I had dropped an egg on the floor and I was being beaten by my mother's shoe.

"YOU LITTLE FUCKING CUNT!" she accused.

"YOU DID THIS ON PURPOSE YOU LITTLE BITCH! Get the fuck out of my sight before I kill you, YOU FUCKING CUNT! I hate you!"

My heart sinks. I remember those mornings and those words ringing in my ears swollen from being punched. It was as if the flood gates had been opened and for the first time I felt what I should have felt for all of those years. I felt angry instead of guilty. I felt validated but violated too.

Child Abuse Barbie

Depression is like drowning in a pool of water, surrounded by everyone you love and them never lifting a finger to help

Bipolar Barbie

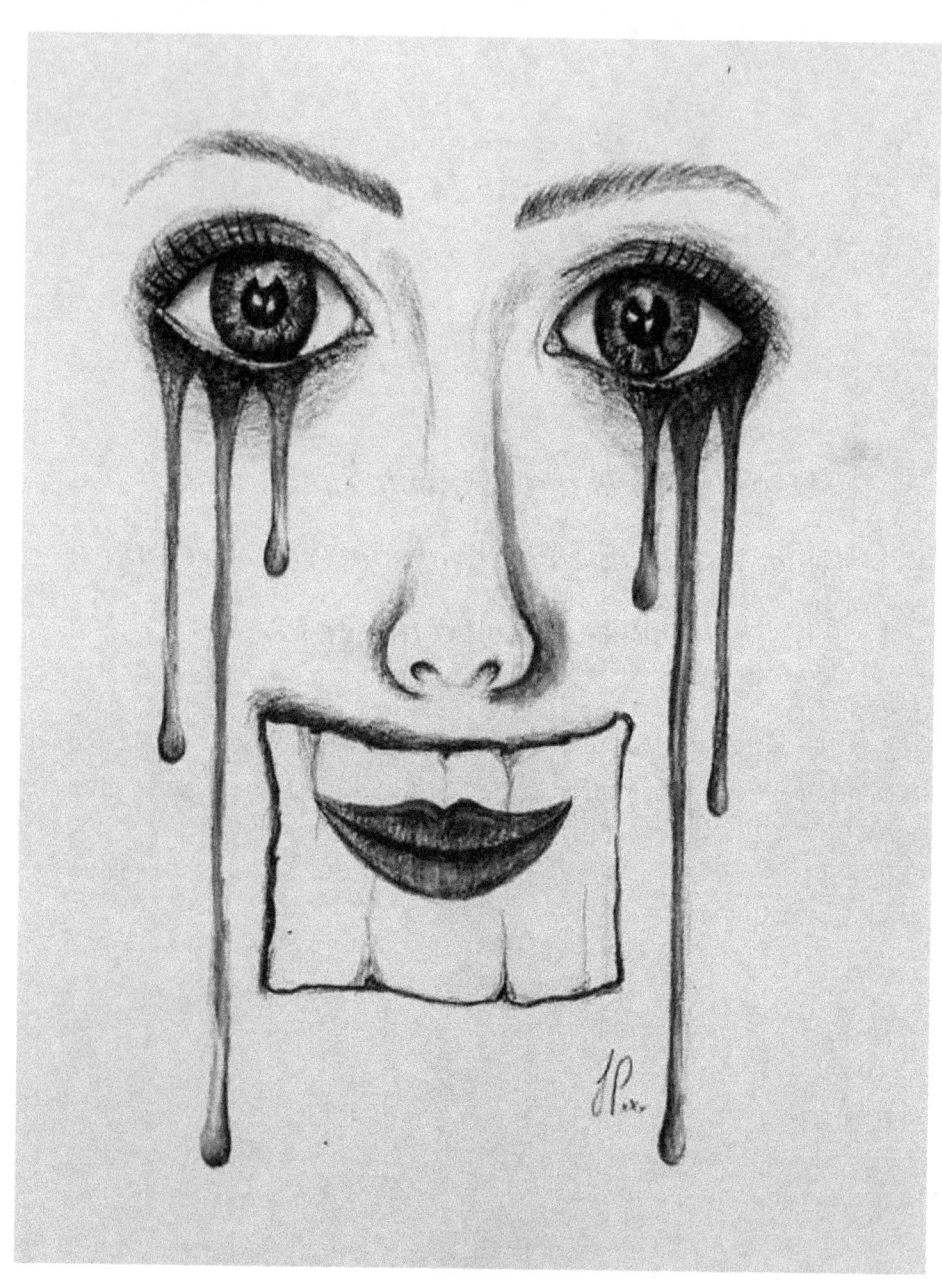

Dear Diary,

Today I told my dad that I have been diagnosed with depression and anxiety. He didn't want to believe it. But he didn't have much choice at this point. He tried to talk to me about it. I could tell he didn't know what to say when I said the words, "I'm depressed." There were so many other things that went unsaid before and after that sentence.

Finally we had some common ground. He had recently been diagnosed with depression and anxiety too. So he is now an expert on the subject. I felt sorry for him. He was trying his best to act like he knew how this whole thing would go down; but there is no way he understood the weight of my situation.

I told him I had been put on medication. He proceeded to tell me that he didn't think that was the right choice. He began to educate me in the ways a person can deal with anxiety. He told me I just need to take deep breaths, calm down and think happy thoughts. He thought he could relate to everything going on in my life. But he couldn't. I was mad. Mad and sad all at the same time.

An argument ensued. It wasn't heated. Just more a clashing of opposing opinions. He was frustrated with me because I wouldn't take his advice. I was upset because he wouldn't listen to me. He hung up on me. It hurt.

Tears are streaming down my face right now. I am devastated that my hero is abandoning me in my time of need. Why did daddy not want to save his little girl? I wanted him to drive to campus and take me home. I wanted him to care enough to take care of me. I didn't care if I was in trouble. I didn't care if he dragged me home by the ear kicking and screaming. I just wanted him to be there.

I was so upset because he wouldn't listen to me. I felt alone. I felt embarrassed and I felt afraid.

No one believes me when I tell them that I am not okay. People are not afraid to tell me that something is wrong with me but they don't care why. Tears are streaming down my face right now as I'm writing this; the pain is overwhelming, unbearable even. But *why?* Why did daddy abandon me in my time of need?

He hung up on me! It hurt so much – like someone stabbed a knife straight into my chest and left it there. For a long time after, I sat in my room, completely ignoring the world around me. I was furious! I wanted to punch something and scream! But really I know that I am just devastated and disappointed. I reverted back to that little girl feeling cold and alone. Abandoned by her hero.

My tears were unstoppable as they streamed down my cheeks while I was sobbing uncontrollably onto my pillow. I know he didn't speak these exact words but the translation was clear. Dad didn't care that his baby girl was in pain.

Finally, when I got up from bed, it took everything inside of me not to scream every swear word I knew at the top of my lungs. I didn't because what good would it do? It wouldn't get the attention of the one person I needed it to.

I now know that to be alone is a fate worse than death.

Ignored Barbie

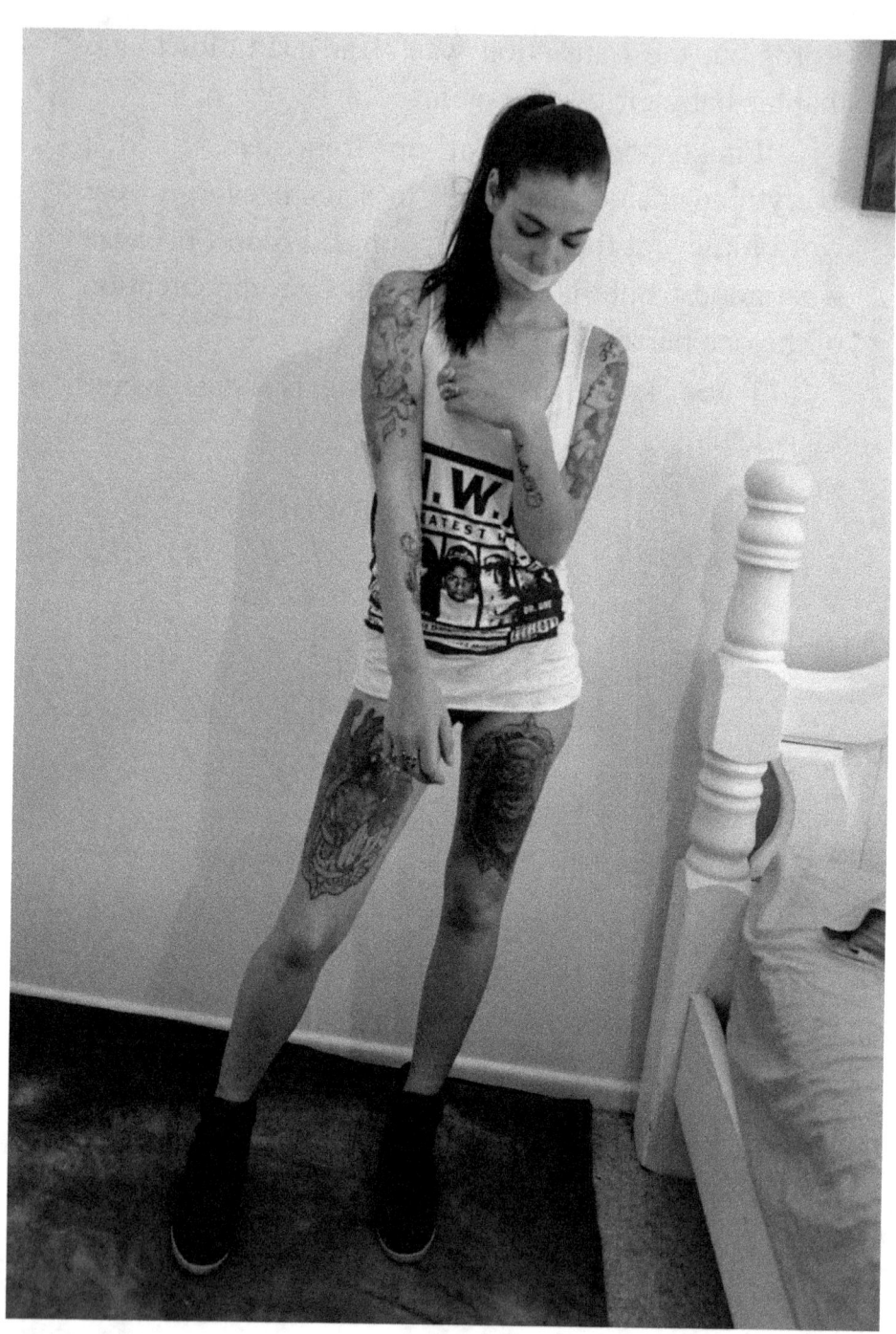

Dear Diary,

If you could see me right now, you would notice a lot of blank expressions, gazing off into the distance, not listening, not coping, laying down in the shower, laying down in bed, laying down anywhere really. It is a lot of 'head in hands' contemplating this dilemma. It is swimming through the depths of despair struggling to breathe. But all of this is silent and mostly private. You won't see me lying on the floor contemplating what I have to live for, trying to balance the scales to find reasons to stay alive. You won't see the cogs ticking over in my mind wondering what troubles today may have in store.

I am removed from my body as I slide down the slopes of depression towards suicide. The worse I get, the less present I am. Maybe it's my body's way of dealing with the incredible pain. Maybe it zones me out so I don't have to experience the excruciating reality of this traumatic existence. Maybe it's a coping mechanism so my body doesn't go into shock. Or maybe this is me going into shock? All I know is that each day I lose more and more time.

I don't know where I go. I find myself stirring a cup of tea for fifteen minutes. I get in my car and find myself sitting in the car park at work forty-five minutes later. I was crying; the tears were sliding down my face in a never-ending stream of sorrow.

People constantly catch me doing something I didn't even know I was doing. There's a disconnect between my consciousness and my body. I can touch my physical body but I can't control it.

I realised I was in the shower this morning after an hour when the water was running cold. I don't even remember waking up. I found myself curled up on the hard tiles like I had passed out there the night before. I didn't even realise I was doing it 'til then. Where do I disappear to?

I almost ran off the road yesterday in the same disconnected state. I was driving and just wasn't there. *Where do I go?* I don't know. But as I sink deeper into depression, it happens more and more. The longer it goes on, the worse it gets. It is like falling down a never-ending mine shaft. I find myself just sinking down to the floor and "waking up" ages later wondering why my body feels like it's paralysed. Why can't I move? It's like my brain isn't connected to my body. All the neuronal signals are mixed up. It's like all of these neurons in my brain, they're not responding to what I want them to do. It used to be easy-peasy for me, but now it feels like everything is so hard!

My eyes are an ocean of dry tears. My mind a sea of unspoken thoughts. I want to cry but I can't let go. I fear letting the dam break.

I imagine myself sinking to the bottom of the

ocean and pretend someone is coming to rescue me. But I fear it's too late. I am tired, exhausted and unsure how long I can continue letting myself sink. I have given up trying to swim. I am just floating awaiting something else to determine my fate. I imagine losing consciousness as the cold agonizing water makes contact with my skin. Sinking like the titanic suddenly realising that drowning is inevitable. I am losing the battle against my mind and I am coming to terms with the end. I am weighed down by my dread adrift all alone.

 I don't know how much more of this I can take! I just want to disappear. I want to be gone. I want this all to stop! But how? How can I escape this misery? Why can't I go back? Why can't I return to what I once was?

Dissociation Barbie

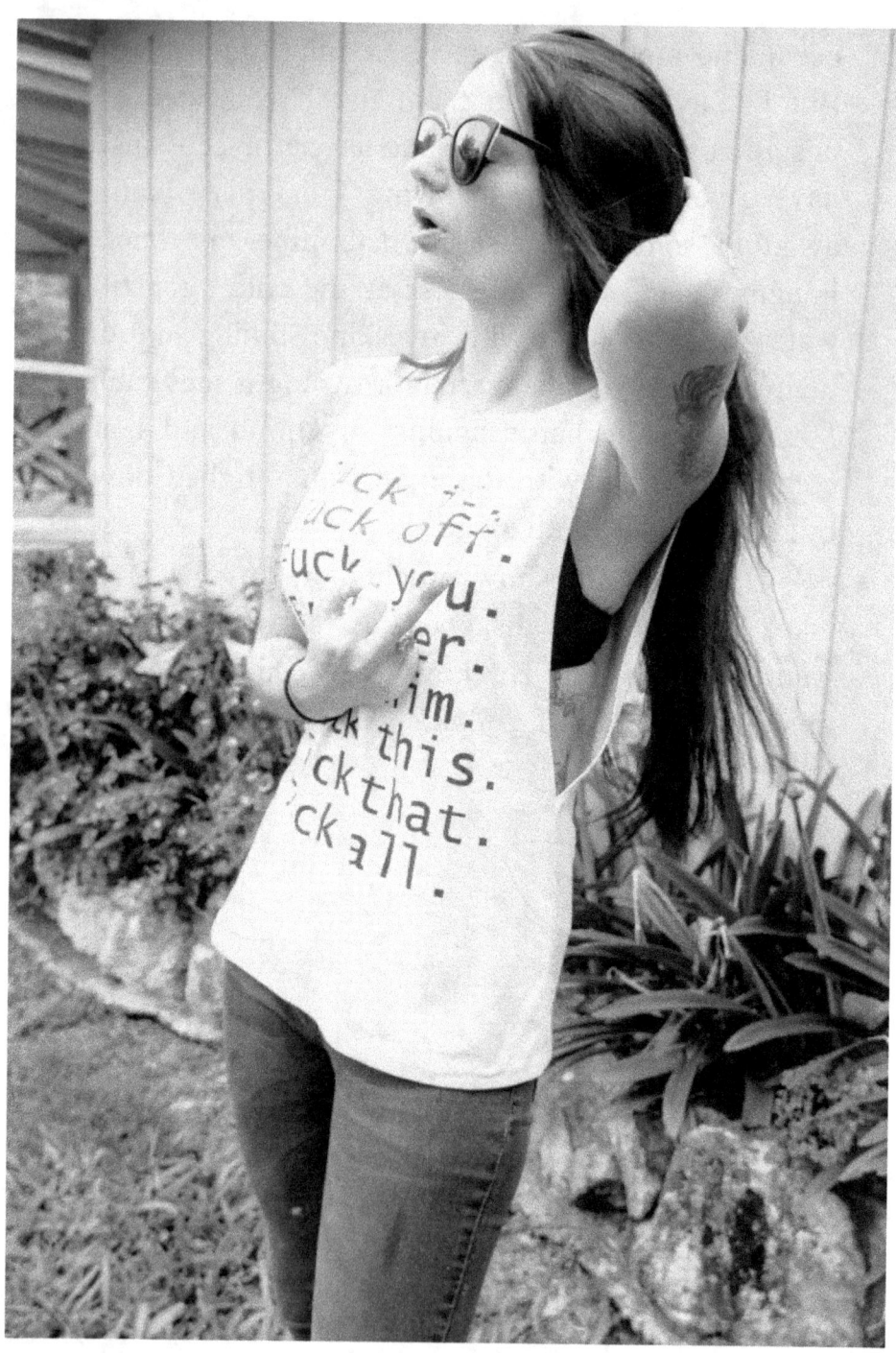

Dear Diary,

I am in tears. They are streaming down my face and soaking into the paper as I write. Splashing onto the pages like a downpour of torrential rain. I am afraid I will start a great flood, drown in my room as well as my sorrows. Why am I so sad? Because I can not believe what just happened.

I have had quite the day. I spent all morning at uni jumping from office to office discussing my situation with professors and student advisers. I barely scrapped by last semester and this one has begun even worse. I see no version of my future where I will be able to pull of the same miracle I did just last semester. At the time I was functioning on pure Adrenalin and manic energy, but my magic has run out. No amount of determination will save me now, my mojo has run out.

Every person I spoke to on campus listened to me intently and responded with empathy and selfless sincerity. They were understanding of my situation and showed compassion towards my pain, despite barely knowing me. Some had known me a mere few weeks and others met me on this day. I felt comforted and like for the first time in a long time I was going to be alright. A weight had been lifted off my shoulders. I had been freed from the expectation that I must maintain a full study load and work full time to support myself while battling with my brain to stay alive. The absurdity of my current situation had been brought to my attention. Apparently working while studying was like having two full time jobs and the expectation to somehow achieve high marks in all aspects of my studies and life whilst maintaining a constant smile and state of togetherness was unrealistic.

I felt understood and at ease for the first time in a very long time. That was until I called my mother to let her know that I would be deferring my studies while I recovered from my recent surgery and stint in hospital. I declared that I would be taking a semester to gather myself, heal and hopefully find the will to live again. I informed her that my mind was consumed with suicidal thoughts and there was simply no way I could continue living this way. I was way past breaking point and something had to give. I either died or put my dreams on hold to catch my breath. I needed time to figure out what was going on and what living with diagnosed depression and anxiety really meant.

She listened for the minute it took me to speak. I heard silence on the other end of the line until I finished and she broke it like a truck smashing through a carnival.

"How could you do this to me?!" she shouted with spite. I was perplexed by the accusatory tone and anger in her voice.

"How dare you do this to me?!" she repeated with swelling rage.

I was confused and lost for words so she kept on speaking.

"What am I going to tell me friends at the gym now?"

"How could you embarrass me like this?"

"How do you think this is going to make me feel when I have to tell them my daughter is a law school drop out?!"

She burst into tears and the sobbing faded off into the distance. I was in shock.

My sisters voice broke the silence as she got on the phone and asked me what I had done to make mum cry? Before I could respond she abused me for hurting our mothers feelings and then huffed as she hung up. My mothers wailing in the distance was abruptly cut off and I was left in stunned silence with my phone in my hand. That was certainty not how I thought that conversation was going to go.

I am in disbelief. Out of the two points I made: deferring University for a Semester and telling my mother I was suicidal, I thought for sure the latter would be the take away from the conversation.

I felt twenty percent confused and seventy nine percent abandoned. I was only one percent angry. I didn't know whether that anger was towards myself or her. The last thing I wanted was to make anyone else upset. I guess I was wrong for thinking that even for a minute my family would care about me enough to actually listen to what I was going through.

Abandoned Barbie

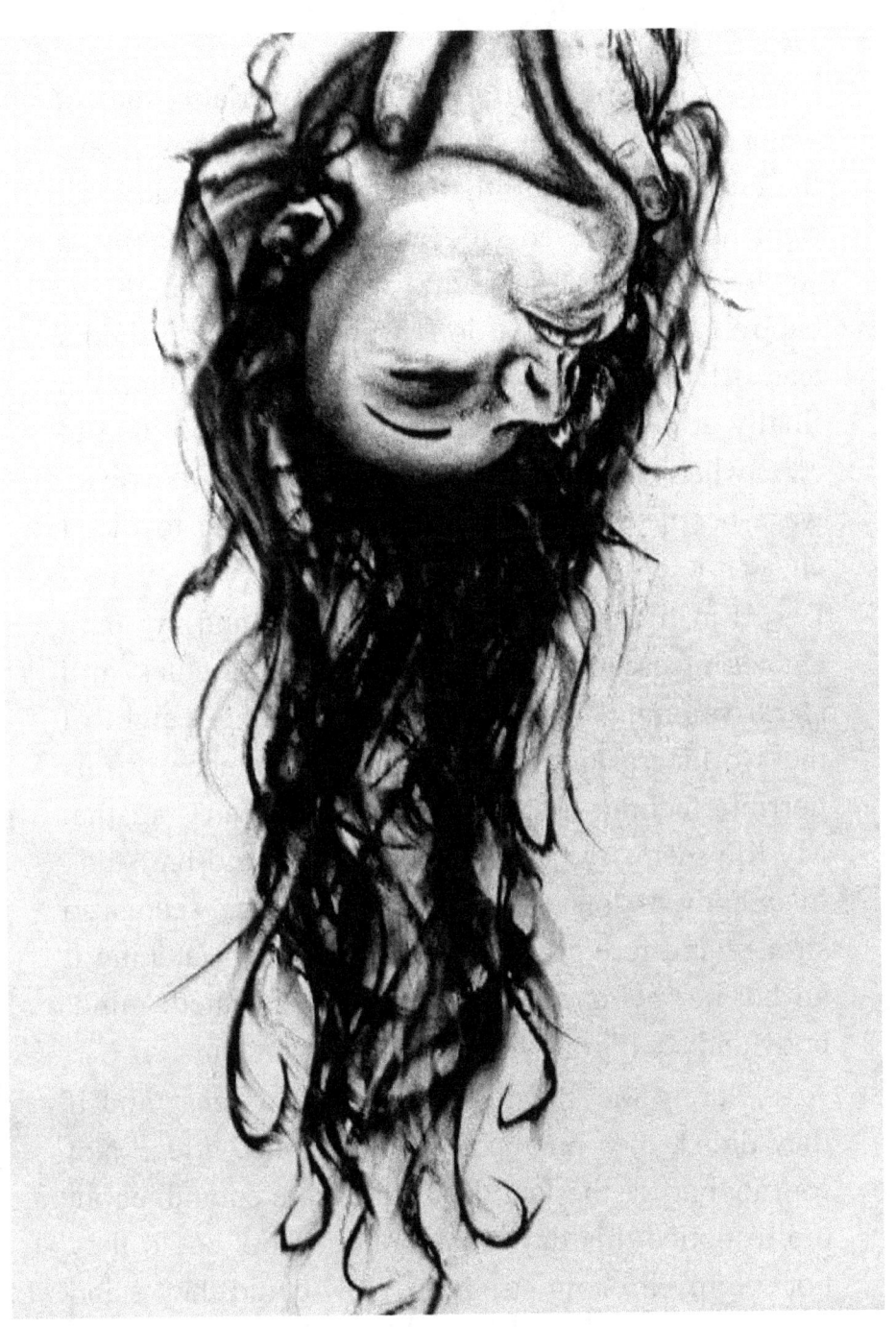

Dear Diary,

As I lay on the floor of my shower after the hot water runs cold, contemplating whether or not I have the energy to pick up that razor blade and end it all right now, I realised I never really thought about a suicide note. But I guess all I want is for people to be happy that I'm gone. I don't want anybody to shed a tear. All I would want them to know is that I'm finally at peace. I've fought too hard for too long to care what happens after I'm gone. I do, however, want people to know that I didn't choose to die, I chose not to live like this anymore.

I'm living in this violent prison, and my only chance of escape is through suicide. I'm stuck in a spiral spinning faster and faster with the weight of the world crashing down. I am consumed by this horrible feeling. It smothers me, and I can't breathe. My life seems to belong to a stranger, and I'm stuck in a body I don't recognise. Everything seems so strange and foreign. I am outside myself watching it all but not being able to help. I am defeated; mind, body and soul. You win depression, you win.

Surely they all knew the end was near and if they didn't, then maybe they should shed a tear. Not for me, but for the fact they didn't care enough about me to notice this day was coming. How could they not see my lifelong struggle? How could they stand by and watch me suffer without lending a hand?

Saying "I don't want to hear about your depression," is like confirming you want to be notified of my death.

    I don't blame them though. Maybe they didn't know how to be there for me? I can't help but think about what is worse to imagine. The fact they were so self-absorbed they didn't know or that they knew and still didn't do anything?

Help Me Barbie

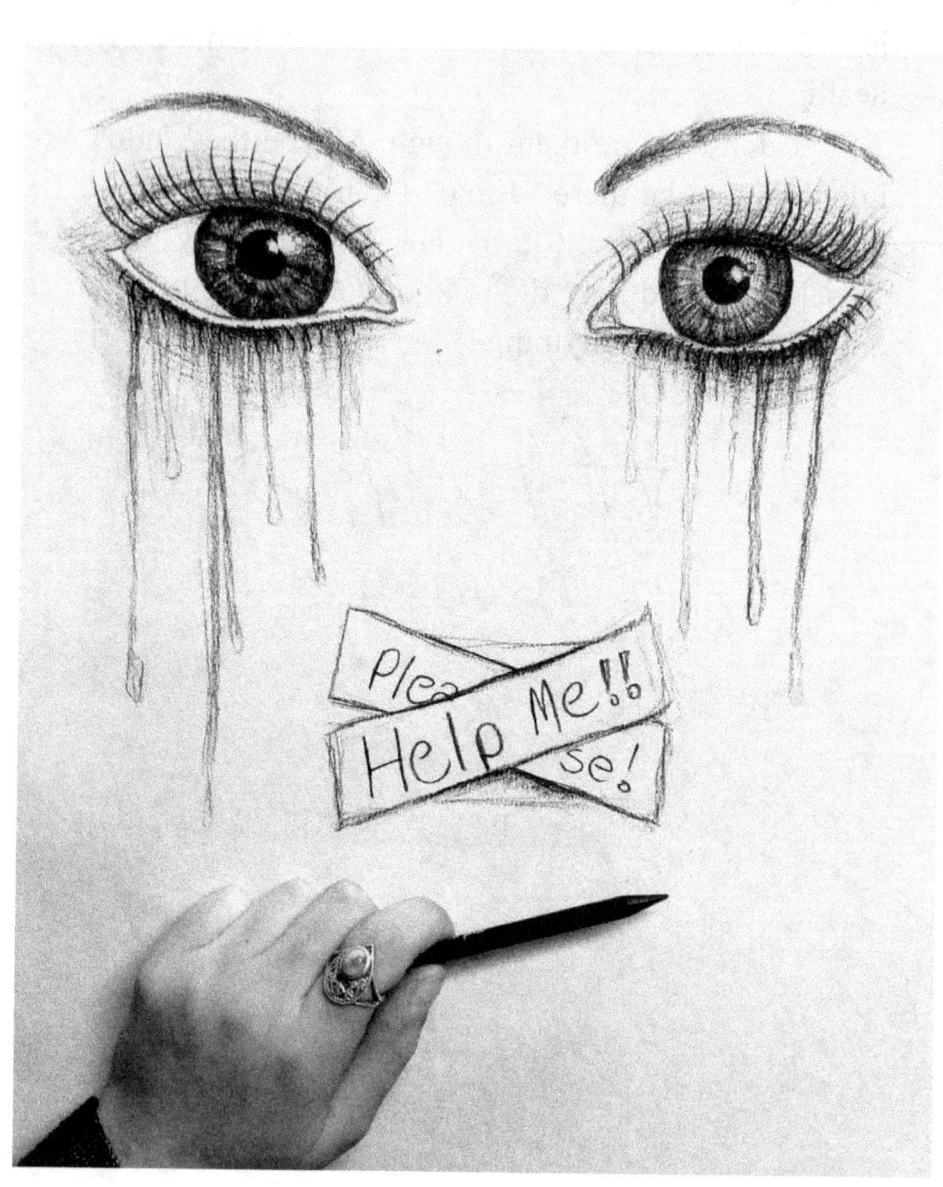

Dear Diary,

I feel like I'm always running but with nowhere to go. Sometimes I'm so alive I feel like I'm a rock star dancing to the beat of my own song or starring in my own Broadway show. I am living in a never-ending episode of *The Bold and the Beautiful*. I am an actor being directed off a script I have never read. Each scene is a surprise, yet I get a strange sense of Déjà vu every time.

These days of my life disappear with the intensity in which they arise. I find myself more often than not screaming for help, and nobody seems to hear a thing. My screams make as much of an impact as a single drop of rain in the ocean. My tears come and go like the ocean tides too. But my sadness is a secret that I hide from nearly everyone in my life. But why? I don't want to lie. I want to speak the truth. I even scribbled it on my arm today. "HELP!" That four letter word that doesn't seem to roll off the tongue and when it does, it always seems to fall on deaf ears anyway.

I have no other choice but to take my pain and direct it at myself. I think about the blade gliding over my skin and carving the words I wish I could speak. I cut, not for attention, but to make a statement. It's my way of declaring that my pain is real. They can still try to deny it, but now it's written in blood. The scars immortalise my pain and suffering. It's a way of screaming "Hey! it's real to me! Now you don't have to acknowledge it. I did it myself."

My clothes are soaked in blood and tears. I cry, and I don't know why. All I know is that everything is not fine. My body's on fire. It's been burning internally; my structures are beginning to collapse. My core is nothing but charcoal and ash. My foundation is shaking and I need to get out! But how do I run from myself?

I am tired of waking up every day already exhausted or not going to sleep at all. I am sick of hoping for the best and doing my best, only to find out it's never good enough. I'm tired of pretending to be okay when I'm not. I'm tired of being told I'm making this all up and being judged. I hate working harder than anyone I know just to survive and be criticised for the way I live my life.

I hate how people ignore the fact that what I choose to do is wake up every day and fight even when I don't want to. To rise to the challenges of another day over and over again despite how much I want to give up. It's hard, with this constant pressure on my shoulders and these thoughts in my head telling me that it'll all be better if I just stop fighting for a while. But no matter how much pain there is, or how many times life knocks me down, somehow I always find a way back onto my feet and keep going.

I am like the Rocky Balboa franchise. Somehow I always make a comeback. I know the ocean is swallowing me whole, but I am not afraid. It has become my new home and I can't escape it now. The only thing left to do is make peace with it before my time runs out.

Self-Harm Barbie

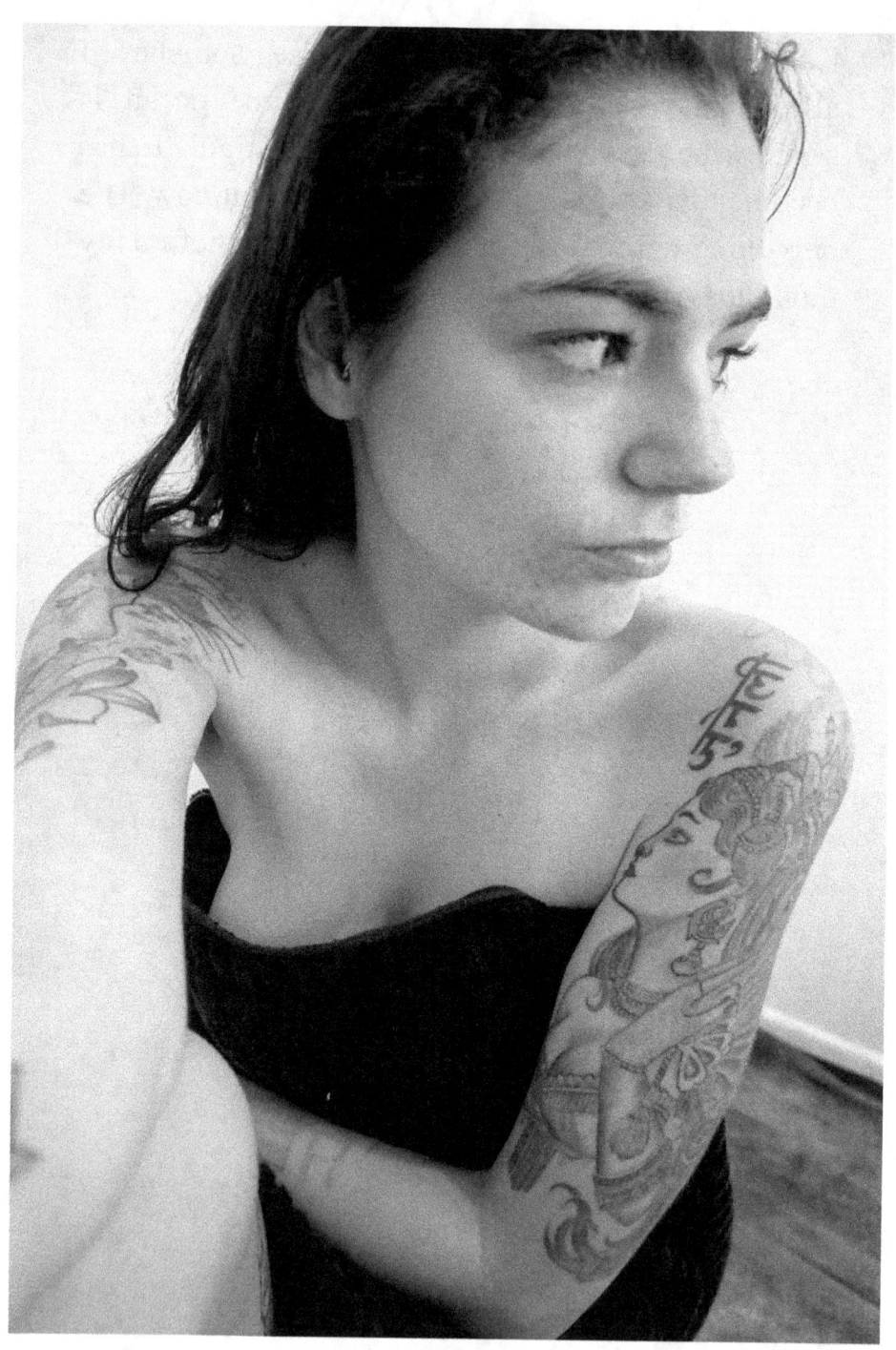

Dear Diary,

Do you know what it feels like to be made of lead? To have sadness exist in your soul, festering like a cancer you can't control? For your heart to beat for a reason, you can't seem to find. To dive into the waters of hell with your head hung low, wading through the depths of despair trying to find a way out of a place no one claims exists? No one comes searching for you because they don't believe you are lost. You're looking for a world that seems so far away, maybe one you have never known. Living in a place that doesn't feel like home, existing in a body that is not your own. Crippled by a power no one understands. Fighting every minute of your life to keep yourself afloat in the dangerous seas of mental illness. No land can be seen on the horizon, no lifeboat is around.

People pass you by, gawk and stare but never lend a hand. They watch you drown. *Why,* you ask? Because they don't think you need saving. Do you know what it feels like to not be worthy of a saviour? To come to the conclusion after years of reaching out that you are alone in this fight and if you don't save yourself no one will? To then try and fail to the best of your abilities; to be stuck in a corpse that wants to return to its grave but a soul that wishes to fly up to heaven? To fight a war, you can't seem to win and worse still no one believes you are in? My plight is ignored, my fight undermined with suggestions, advice and useless opinions about how to win a war a minute ago they denied existed? Experts of the unknown, the strange and bizarre; they give it to you for free but warn you can end your own suffering if you just believe there was nothing wrong with you, to begin with.

It's not like they know what it feels like to have their brain feel like an actual battlefield where every thought is attacking itself with a knife or gun until there's nothing left of them but dead space. They don't know how hard it is to live when you can't even function properly because your thoughts are spinning in circles around themselves, never stopping long enough for anything productive to occur before something bad happens and they start all over again. Braver warriors have lost this fight. Their struggles are silent and their deaths misunderstood.

All it takes is for us to accept that this war exists to give our soldiers back their reason to fight. To give them hope that what they fight for is real and that it exists. To make it attainable for all!

Warrior Barbie

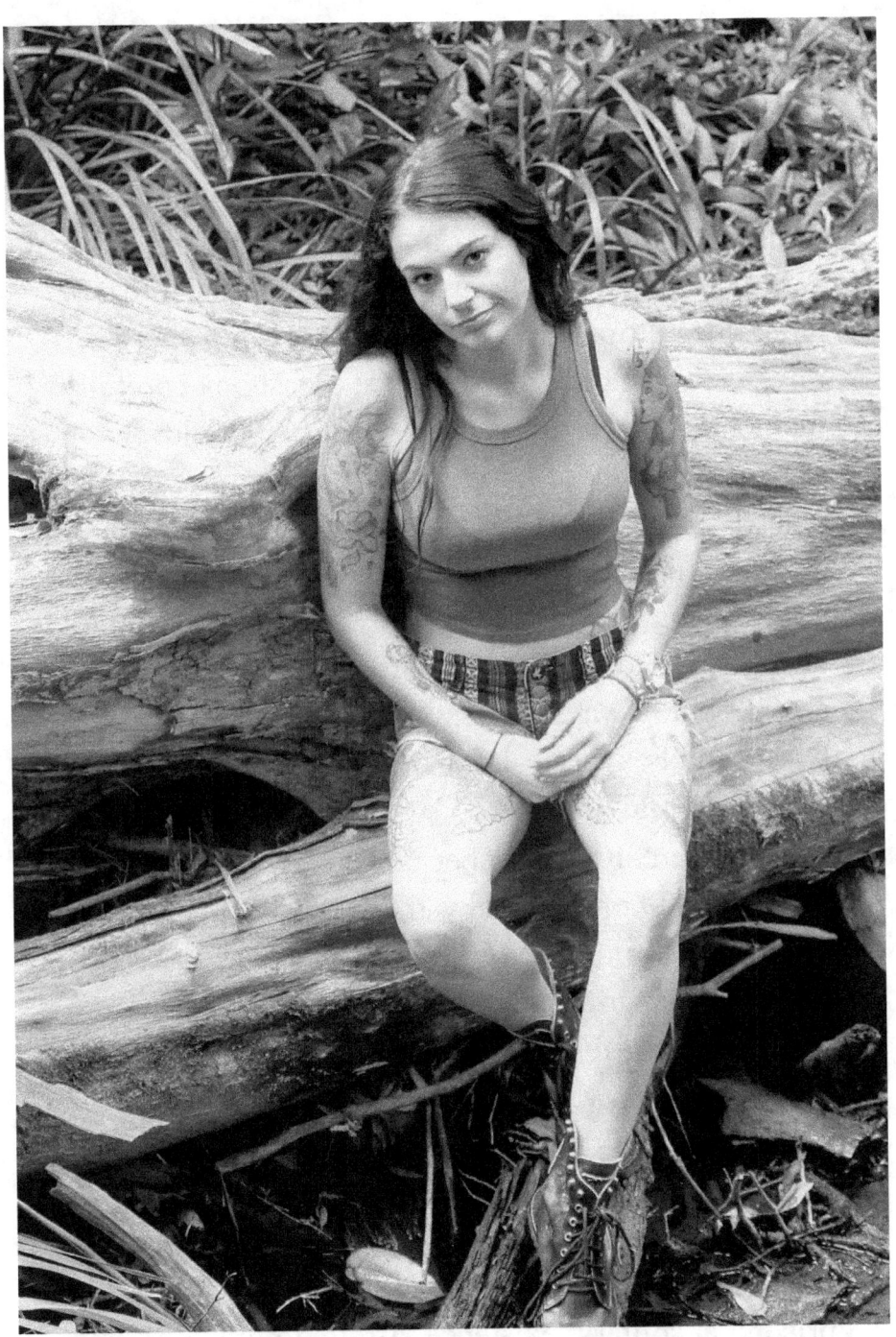

Dear Diary,

    I looked back today and remembered a time when I felt whole. A time when I actually enjoyed being alive. I've felt the opposite for so long it's hard to imagine there was ever a time I actually felt alive. A time I could walk through life without the threat of landmines blowing up in my face. A time where my mind was more roses or at least a carefully manicured lawn instead of this battlefield. Even remembering those happy times makes me sad. Oh, what I would give to be back in that time. But alas … I have nothing to give. Chasing my sanity is like a dog chasing its tail. More likely than not a fruitless endeavour. Running around in circles determined to get it, but always just slightly out of my reach. Occasionally I get a hold of it, but I lose it faster than I can find it.

    I scarcely remember a time when I wasn't trapped and constricted by the burdens and fears of my mind. A time where I wasn't wrapped in barbed wire, torn apart with every move. Nowhere is safe. A time when life was worth living, and people were kind. A time when I was ignorant of the daily struggles I now face. A time when I really could achieve the dreams I wanted to achieve. Now they just seem like fantasies lost in space as I pace around the room I have not left in weeks. Confined to this prison; a solitary existence afraid to live. A time when wanting to take my own life had never crossed my mind. A time when I believed people were friendly before I learned most are hostile.

I took so much for granted. The ease of brushing my teeth or going to the beach. Having a life full of eager ambition. Now failure seems like a tradition. A time when I believed true love meant doing everything and anything for the ones you love. A time I felt safe and protected around those I hold close to my heart. I did not believe anyone would willingly punish me for being who I am. The betrayal stings with all of my being. I guess that's just my opinion. I believe in treating others how you wish to be treated and expect others to do the same as a simple courtesy. I was wrong.

I wish to return to a time I felt like I belonged in this world. When wrong or right seemed black or white. When life gives you lemons, they say make lemonade. Easier said than done but life has given me a lot of horrible things, and lemons are not one of them. A time when I thought everyone had a voice, that a person could never feel this much hurt. A time I could never imagine ending up like this. A time when I thought the people I loved would be there for me when I really needed help but alas I was a naive fool. Nobody does anything unless it suits them.

A time when I wasn't alienated from everyone I cared about, but then again in a way I always was. I just didn't know it yet. A time when people didn't talk behind my back, a time when people didn't call me lazy to my face. A time my family didn't roll their eyes at me when I told them I couldn't work and they'd reply, "can't, or *won't*?". A time my heart didn't break every time someone told me I was making it all up. That it was my choice to be like this. That their struggles were the same as mine if not more significant. But because they just deal with it and get on with life, I should too. Implying that I actually can.

A time when there wasn't a time limit on sympathy or even tolerance. Just this morning I was given advice, oh how I hate that! "You need to just get it together, work on yourself for god's sake!" What the fuck do they think I do all day? I guess they observe me doing very little, but they are completely unaware of all that I deal with even when lying still. I can't stress how counterproductive it is when I'm trying to convince myself I am enough, I can do this when it's clear I can't, and then someone belittles all my efforts with a simple sentence.

The stigma is ripe, and it hurts. It does make me want to end my life. Why bother trying when I'm getting nowhere? Why bother trying when I am condemned for my efforts? Because deep down I want to win even if everyone else makes out I am deliberately trying to lose. When people make out I do this for a reason I am yet to comprehend. Why would I do this to myself? What do you think I get out of this? "Oh, how nice it must be you; to not work, to not leave your house, to sit around distracting yourself with Netflix and not socialise." Do you think I enjoy being like this? Do you think this is the life I would choose for myself if I had a choice?

The saddest part is people actually do. Nearly everyone. You are all naive ... I do not enjoy one second of being like this! Life is hard enough to live. This battle is tough enough on its own. Don't be the asshole that makes out I've done this to myself. Because you will only confirm that I am in this fight alone. Maybe I am alone, maybe I have done this to myself. But I'd rather be alone than around people who constantly make me feel lonely.

Why am I scared of people, my psych asks me? Well besides the fact I've learnt the hard way I cannot trust anyone not to cause me pain and hurt me (even the ones I love)? There's the fact that no one understands. No one gets it, no one even tries! No one believes me, no one accepts that my struggles are real, and any person who comes across me in my mentally ill state makes it their civic duty to put me down, to tell me I'm faking it, to tell me I'm making it all up, to tell me everything I am sure you have all heard before. Not ONE person has ever made me feel otherwise. So yeah, people suck.

Quite frankly I am more terrified of people than I am of being mentally ill the rest of my life because every human interaction I have triggers long-lasting wounds to open up and bleed profusely. Nowhere is safe. I am cut to shreds walking through life being torn apart by wolves and vultures and they all just look at me like "what the hell are you doing? Pull your shit together!" If only they could see my wounds ... although I am convinced it wouldn't help because they just don't want to believe that such evil can exist in this world.

How can a person want to die when our sole purpose is to live? I don't think you ever understand that until you have suffered for so long that being alive is the most intense pain you have ever known. Death would be a mercy. Like in the movies when someone is being tortured, and they beg for their aggressors to kill them. Well ... that's exactly what I have felt like for as long as I can remember. I've been begging for mercy for years. No one wants to hear it because they simply can't see my torment. Or is it just that they just don't bother to look?

Invisible barbie

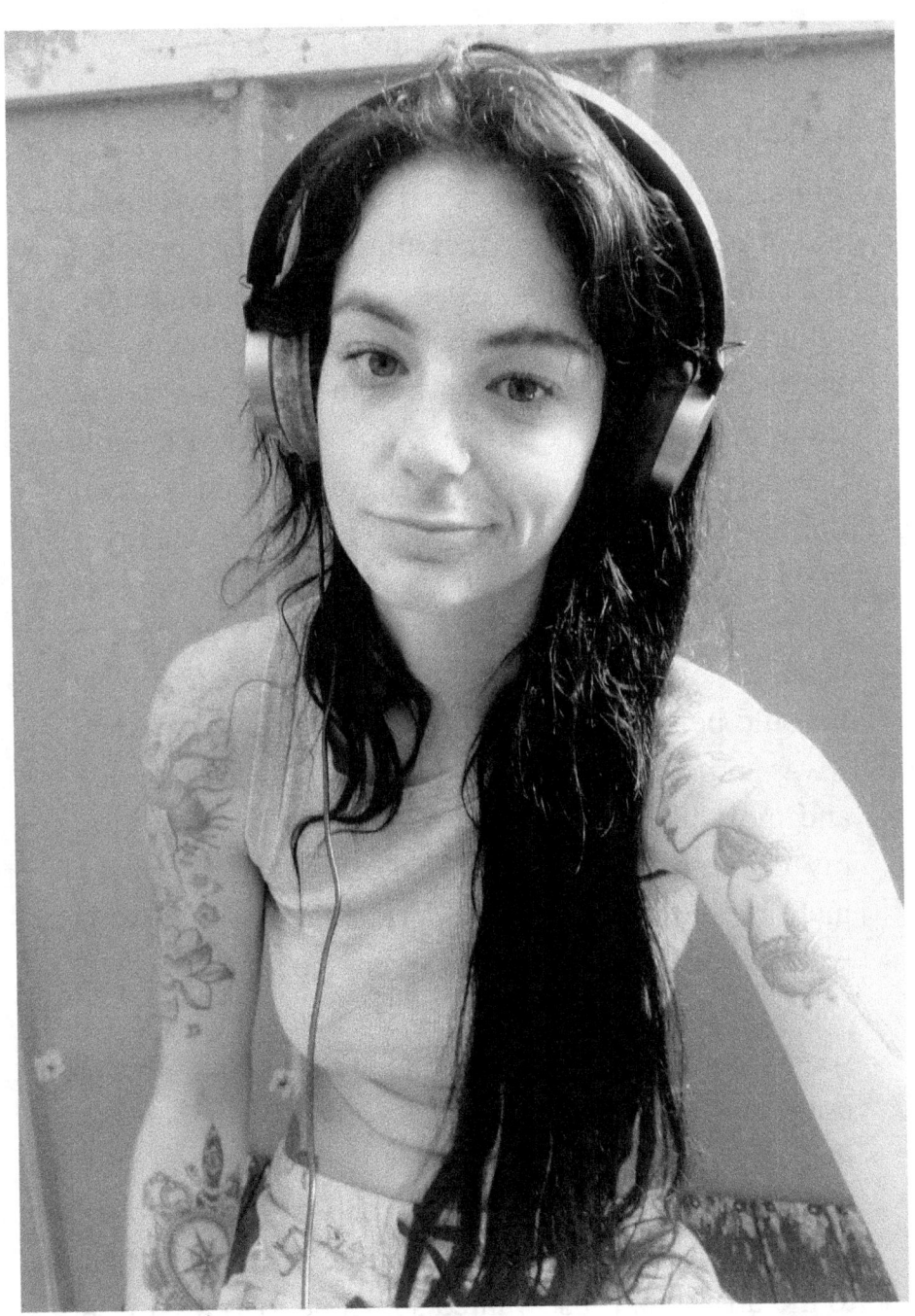

Dear Diary,

Yesterday I wanted to kill myself. I have thought about trying to kill myself for the better part of most of my life, but yesterday I was pretty close. I felt hopeless, alone and that all the fantastic people I have in my life weren't enough, which made me feel guilty. I was also angry that no one could help me, not even myself. I contemplated the various ways of doing it. I am thankful that I am terrified of heights because that's the only sure fire way I could think of doing it. I had the pills I needed. But unfortunately, I have learned from personal experience the trick is getting them to stay in your stomach long enough to work. I have done that enough times before to realise I would be vomiting my guts up in more agony than I was in now by sunrise. I knew it was a tricky one and most likely wouldn't work. I also knew driving my car into a tree would also allow for a massive margin for error. I was smart enough to know it would probably do more harm than good.

I held on. I tried to ignore the monster screaming inside my head. He was heating up my body and boiling my blood. I could feel it burning through my veins. The pain was building as I slumped over and wished for a better life. I was searching for just a glimmer of hope as I reached out to the universe. I just wanted someone to know I was hurting. It's easy to think no one cares when no one knows. I know there must be people out there that care. I just wish they told me once in a while. People ask me if having tens of thousands of fans on social media make me want to live more. I wish it did. Their support is fantastic and fabulous. But when the people closest to you, the people you care about most, the ones that are expected to care don't … It hurts so much more.

The most vital thing I did yesterday was reach out. It let others know how I was really feeling and actually gave them a chance to let me know they care. It quietened those voices in my head that said they don't, because it gave me proof they did. I think because of that, I awoke today in a slightly better mood. It was accompanied by a raging headache, but I often get those. They are like a lightning storm brewing in my head. They are ferocious and unforgiving. I know they represent change. My brain chemicals must be shifting in my head. It's acting like it's about to burst. It's like fireworks are going off as my body adjusts to new hormones, new influxes of chemicals and who really knows what else. The little whatchamacallits … the neurotransmitters and neurons are firing like the Avengers heroes fighting off an alien invasion.

A sensitivity to change is what I have been told Bipolar Disorder is. Change is my entire life. My body over and under regulates itself. It cannot adjust to change, so it freaks out, and any form of change can spin me for a loop. Today my good mood lasted until about lunchtime when my headache came back into play and I started to feel down. I slipped back into the same headspace I was yesterday. Today had turned into another bad day ... but I stopped myself there.

"Today was a good day!" I said. I'd had more hours of a normal-ish mood than I'd had in over a month. *Today was a triumph,* I thought. I'd managed to stay positive and fight off this black demon from the time I awoke until about 1pm. I would not let its final defeat mid-afternoon ruin a somewhat pleasant start to my day.

I could sense it coming as it worsened all afternoon. My shoulders started caving in, my headache began brooding, heavy weights were crashing over me, dark clouds were circling, fatigue was setting in, and hopelessness was riding in over the horizon.

I spent most of the night staring off into space. I wanted to disappear and shrink away from people. I wanted more than anything else just to become invisible, unnoticeable and insignificant. I wanted to numb the pain coming over me like a storm. I was unpredictable and inconvenient.

It reminds me of the near-death experience I'd had in Sri Lanka. I was over there working in the orphanages and schools teaching. For the weekend I left the tiny village I was living in and went to the south of Sri Lanka for a beachside holiday. I sat on the beach and watched the calm water, but as a Surf Lifesaver, I noticed a strong undercurrent. Tourists were being swept out to sea; unaware they would struggle to get back in against the strong rip underneath.

    Only a few of us, the stronger swimmers, decided to go into the water. Everything was fine until I tried to get back in. I will never forget the moment I realised I was in trouble. The moment I realised I was swimming and getting nowhere. I had been in the same place for over five minutes despite how rapidly I swam. Panic set in, and as the swell picked up I tried to ride the waves in to propel me towards shore, but as they grew and peaked close to the banks, the monsters crashed down hard on the sand and sucked back twice as strong as they rolled in. Not only was I being pulled under and backwards but the monsters kept rising around me and pummelling me into the sandy, rocky bottom. I was pinned underwater, tossed and turned like I was stuck in a washing machine I couldn't turn off. Gasping for air, I'd reach the surface just as another colossal monster reared his head to pull me under again.

    I remember the desperation kicking in as I

fought against the current. It was the moment I realised I might actually die. Even as a strong swimmer doing my best, it wasn't enough. I understood that sometimes your best wasn't enough. Sometimes no matter how hard you tried you might still get beat. As the clock ticked, my frustration was growing. I could see the shore. The waves were breaking so close to the beach it was only a matter of metres to safety, but no matter how hard I tried I just couldn't get there. I couldn't stand up no matter how close I was. I could almost touch the sand, but it was always just out of my reach. I remember watching all of my friends sipping cocktails on the beach, completely unaware I was choking on water being jammed down my throat.

That was the most terrifying moment of my life to date. I had nightmares about it for months. Every night I'd awake screaming, covered in sweat. "It's over now," I would say, trying to calm my nerves. At least for another night.

I mention it now because I've just realised that the feeling I had on that day on the beach in Sri Lanka before I even knew I had a mental illness is what it all felt like the moment things started to go wrong. The way they have been since that day, never quite getting out of the water. Always being taken with the currents in moods that seem out of my control. The only difference now is that I am not scared. I am so used to this existence I ride the waves as they come and have accepted that at times I will get nowhere. I have accepted that maybe I will never get out of this water. But I will sure as hell fight for my life right up until the day I die.

Drowning Barbie

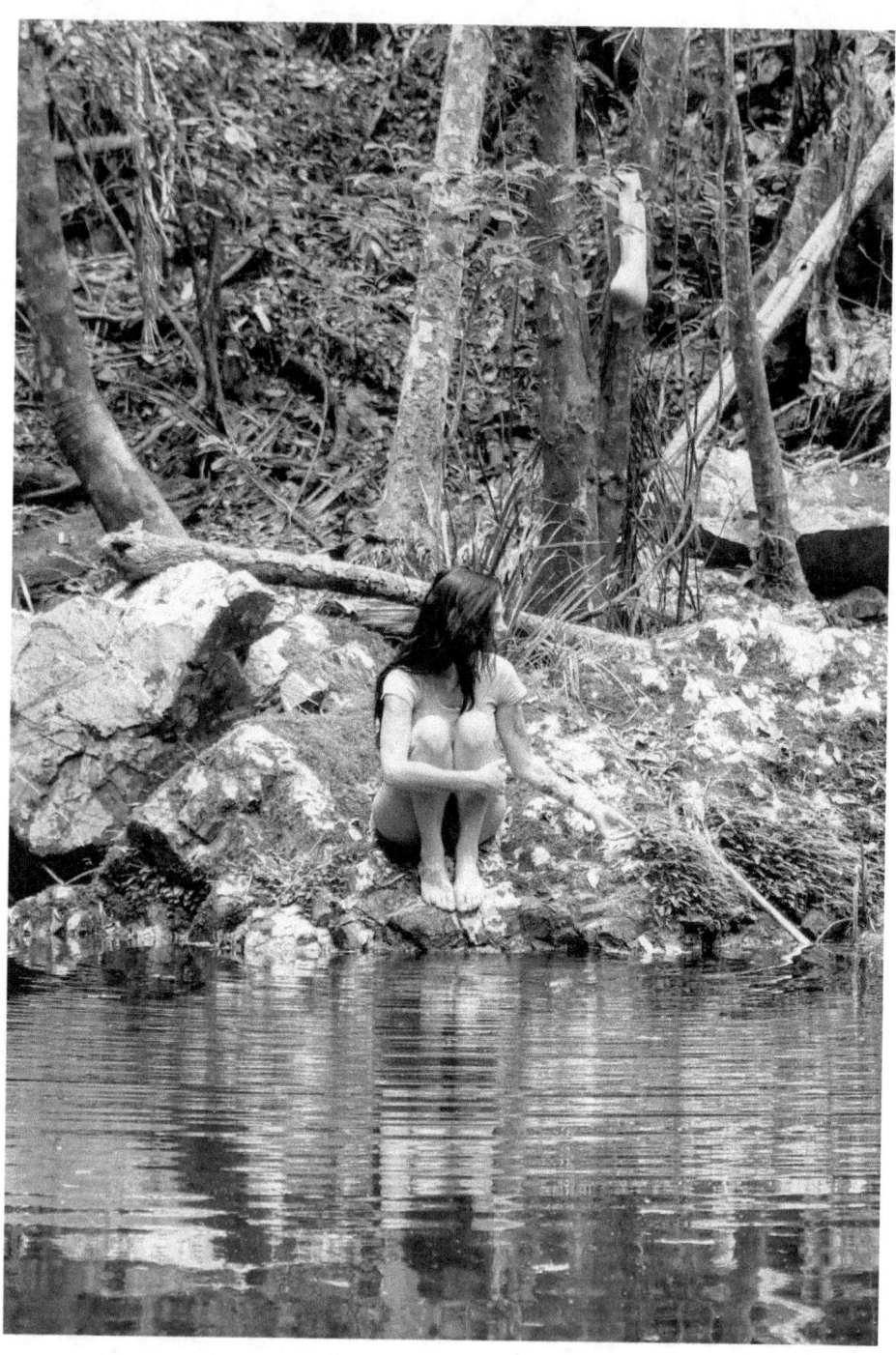

Dear Diary,

    I struggle through the day, shying away from the light; terrified, cold and alone. I'm not even sure why but the weight of the world weighs heavily on my shoulders. If it was literally balanced on my shoulders, I would be Supergirl; I'd be praised for saving the world. Unfortunately that's not the case. It's just my world. So why does it feel so heavy? Why do I feel like the earth is shuddering under my feet? Why do I feel like my chest is going to implode with the weight threatening to crush it? I feel small, yet I want to be smaller. Maybe if I shrink enough no one will find me. Maybe I'll get better at hiding. But it's never enough. I collapse in on myself, as I don't have the strength to hold myself up. I feel my insides churning, flaking off. Piece by piece falling into nothing. I am nothing. It is like falling apart and being squished together all at the same time. My mind wanders in a desert. No particular train of thought or emotion, just heavy as I fall to the floor. I think I'm a bit down today because anxiety has once again reared its nasty head. When my anxiety is high, I feel like my heart is beating out of my chest. My chest is so tight I can't breathe, I feel like I'm being crushed. Distractions are both a nuisance and the best ammunition I've got. Finding the right one in the right moment is tough, and I've tried out many today. Healthy ones. In the past I'd have chosen alcohol or drugs. I shy away from the world partly because I am so vulnerable but also because I don't want to be seen like this.

We are told from a very young age that weakness is a bad thing. It is so ingrained in our society that we are terrified of looking weak in the eyes of others, so we are accustomed to hiding our weaknesses, denying them and pushing them away. Weakness is *not* a bad thing. The only time it is a bad thing is if we don't acknowledge our weaknesses. I spent a large portion of my life suppressing my weaknesses, and they festered inside of me. I began to decay internally because I was so adamant about providing a solid exterior image I neglected myself in the process. People are so determined to hide their weaknesses, so fearful of other people seeing them, that they get extremely angry when someone points them out. Our insecurities then control us.

I was so terrified of acknowledging my faults, even though I knew them well because I had been told my whole life I was defective. I wanted them all to be wrong, so I spent a lifetime trying to prove them wrong in order to show them that I was strong. In doing so, I became weak. Acknowledging our weaknesses isn't what makes us weak, denying them does that. There is incredible strength in knowing your flaws, acknowledging your weaknesses and committing to change them. True strength is knowing you aren't perfect but going on anyway. Even if you know them yourself, pointing them out to others makes you incredibly vulnerable! Some may use them against you and trust me most of them will. But that's only because they are still running around pretending the sun shines out of their ass like they can do no wrong. Dating narcissists really bring this to light. They can do no wrong, they have to constantly preach how perfect they are and manipulate others weaknesses to make them seem strong. But they never leave any room for improvement, so they will never change. In doing so, they are crippling themselves for life. They will always be a disappointment because what people see is only an illusion of what they can never be.

Yet it is those who dare to be vulnerable and flawed, those who dare to show what they are not, those like me who grossly undervalue themselves, that show true strength. To know that you are not perfect, that you are flawed and that you can never amount to the illusions others create makes you incredibly brave. Only when you acknowledge what's wrong and accept your imperfections can you begin to change. Just because you need to work on some things doesn't mean there is anything wrong with who you are as a person. In fact, it might just mean there is everything right.

There's nothing wrong with trying to better

yourself, in fact, we'll all need to do that for the rest of our lives. Most people seek to better themselves in the eyes of others, and to focus on careers, money and possessions. They forget the inward journey that exists as well. Some of the richest people I know have nothing at all.

Our vulnerabilities are what allow us to connect with other people on a deeper level. Only when you let people in to see what's behind the mask, do you open up the possibility to be loved for who you are!

Super Barbie

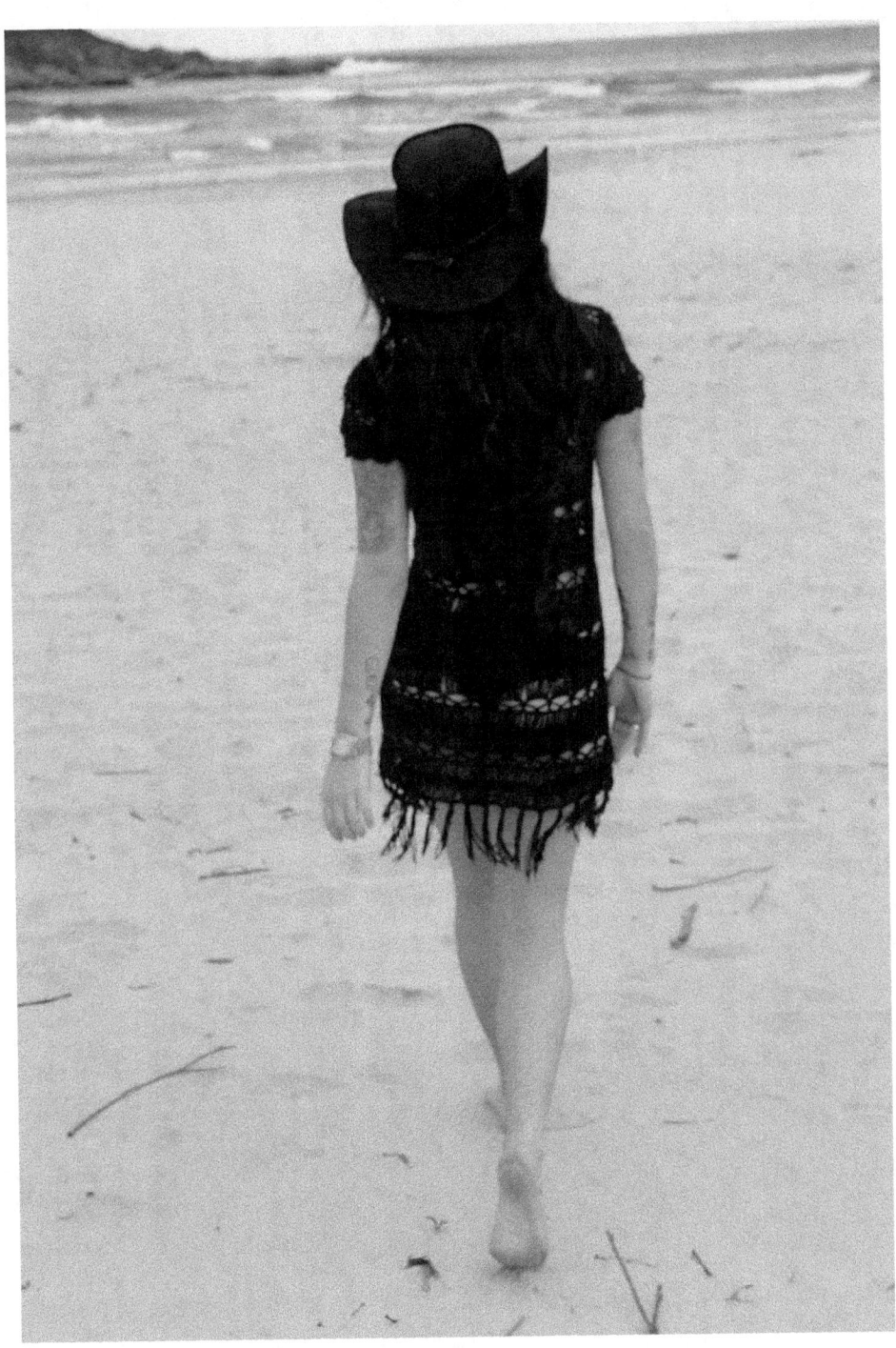

I don't know whether I want to save myself or drown, because I can't seem to do either.

Bipolar Barbie

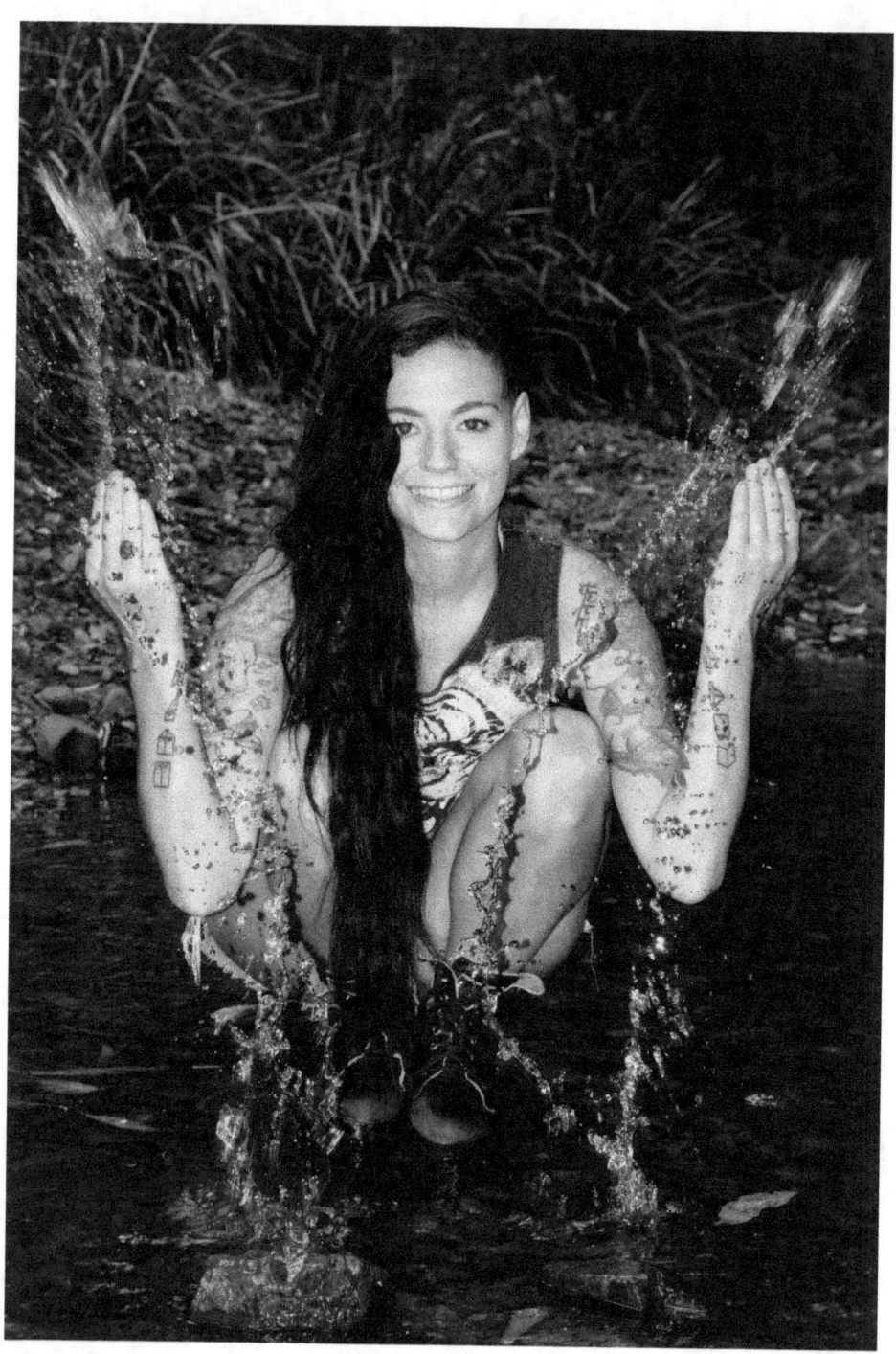

Dear Diary,

My soul screams. I hear it calling my name; it's in excruciating pain. It wants me to set it free. I am screaming inside but walking around like I am barely alive. I am a wax figure with a candle wick burning at both ends. My body is crippled by pain and fear. The devil keeps knocking at my door and I want to yell "I'm not here!" but he has put poison in me, and it's burning me from the inside out. It's like acid melting my stomach lining and leaking into my abdomen. I suffer every second. I have to hide the pain inside. Because no one believes me when I tell them the truth; that just being alive is the greatest pain I know.

I feel it in every cell in my body as depression has taken over. I feel like a lobster being boiled alive. Everything is agony, uncomfortable even lying flat buried deep beneath the covers, but it's the safest place to be. Nothing else can hurt me here.

Lying in bed during the day may be perceived as weak by some. But in fact, it's quite the contrary. I am incredibly strong! I persevere with my skin on fire as I burn from within, the calm on my face is an act of incredible strength. People think I want to lounge around but that is far from the truth. I want to run, I want to hide, I want to disappear, I want to die, none of which I will be lucky enough to have tonight.

I beg someone, anyone, please, end my suffering. I just need it to stop. There's only so long someone can endure such an intense kind of pain. I hide it no longer because I am exhausted. For years I wore it with honour so that the ones I love didn't have to see its true horror. But make no mistake ... words can't describe the thousand types of sorrow I now face.

I am numb, but in agony all at the same time. I can't feel emotion but I can feel pain, and each cell in my body is vibrating, I can't contain this rage. I am trapped inside a cage as I age, afraid to take a bow and leave this stage. I watch my grave being dug. It is like my body is trying to kill itself before the day even starts.

Today is the day I promise myself that I will finally put down my mask. I have lost all the energy to hide the tragedy unfolding within. I can't help but think, here I am in this mess yet again. It's not the first time, and I doubt it will be the last. I just desperately want to find relief from this curse before it strikes again. Another day is done. In the words of Freddie Mercury, "another one bites the dust". My heart is beating so fast I just want to cut it out of my chest and stab it until it dies. Drain my blood until all the poison is out. I dream of simply going to sleep and never wake up every single night.

It feels like I'm walking on hot coals,

surrounded by fire; suffocating from the smoke inhalation as the air in my room ignites. It's like I'm walking around with a plastic bag over my head, or treading water as my body feels like lead. My chest feels empty but it's also being compressed by something heavy. Something is choking me. I can't help but think there's a virus going around. Yet I see everyone else walking about completely unaware or unaffected, and I wish I was them. I am being tortured, burnt alive while everyone else is doing alright.

    I just want it to stop. I'll start begging soon. I don't know what to do. I can't escape it, and I know it's going to hang around for a while. This isn't my first rodeo or round in the ring. I've been boxing this beast for as long as I dare to remember. Never seeming to win, but never being knocked out despite how many times I have been knocked down.

    On this hot summer night I yearn for anything to subdue me, to knock me out. I long to just disappear for a while. I wander the halls of my dorm room wishing to be seen. But everyone else is asleep. I try to creep and sneak around, not daring to squeak or make even a tiny peep. Yet in my head I scream, I run around. I bang on the doors and shout. I want someone to come out. I want someone to find out. See me sitting on the outdoor couch at the break of dawn and reach out. But no one makes a sound.

No one can help me, and I wish they could, but I would never put that burden on them. I suffer in silence because it's the only thing I can do. Help takes a while, a long while and even though I am getting all the help there is, I still find myself in the deepest of suffering.

I want to cry, but my tear ducts are all dried up. I want to scream, but I can't make a sound. I am dying inside, and my thoughts torment me day and night. I just want to sleep all the time because I can't do anything else, but even sleep evades me at this time. I just feel weak and terrified of what is going to happen to me.

There's only so much pain a person can take. Help me. Save me.

It's okay. I'm okay. I hope. That's just it, I will be okay. I don't even know if that is what I want anymore. Maybe I would prefer to drown …? If you can't go up, then you might as well go down.

Rescue Me Barbie

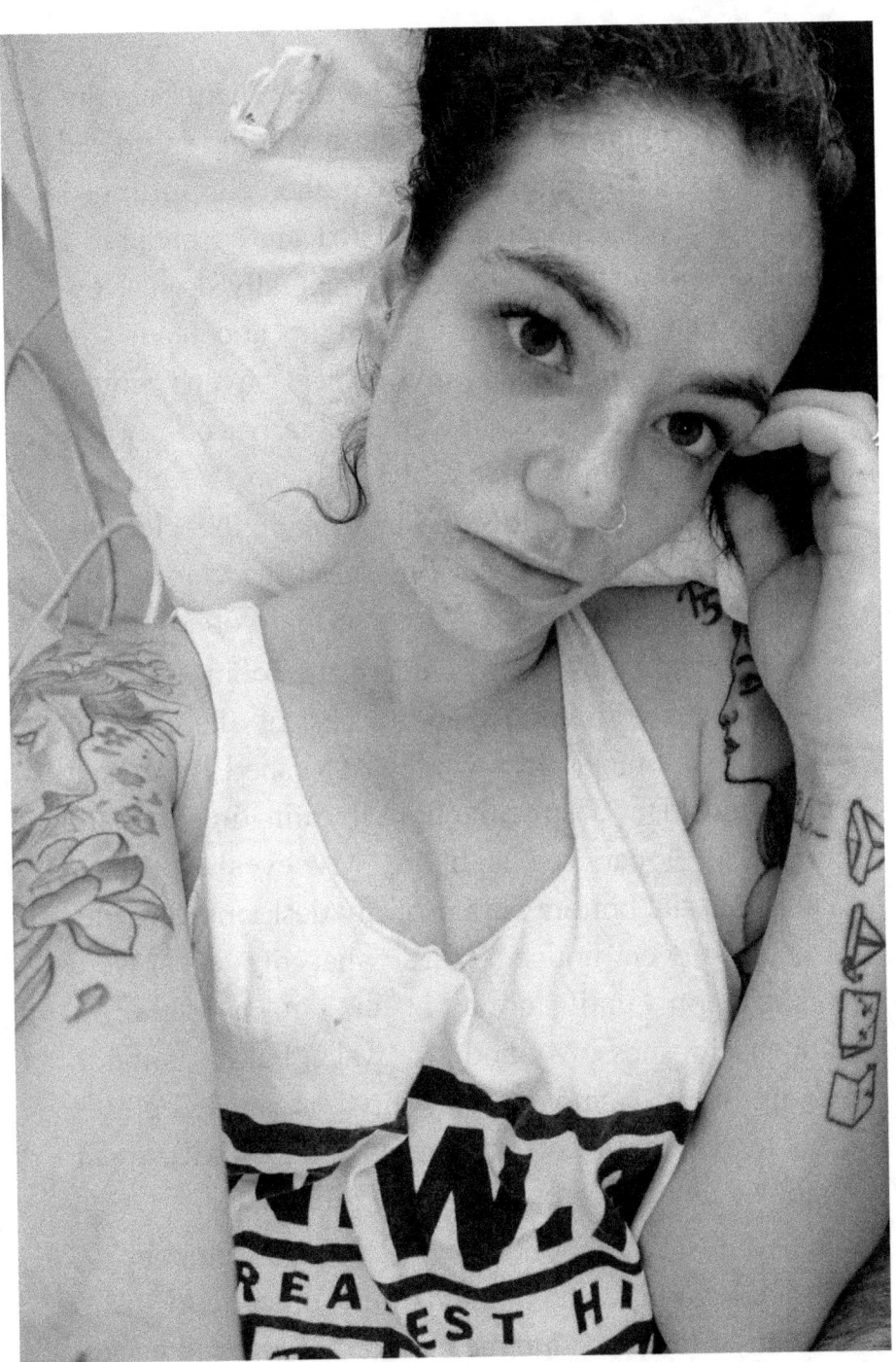

Dear Diary,

I'm alive. It pains me as I write. The thought of sawing through my wrists to cut my veins and bleed out is terrifying, although also rather comforting. I can't help but hate myself for it. I am so pathetic I can't even muster the courage to actually do it. How weak am I? It's now past midnight, and I am still curled up on the floor in my towel. I haven't moved since I got out of the shower. The carpet on my uni dorm room floor is incredibly itchy, so I've made a dirty-clothes-pile-pillow. Even though the cleaners have come through, I can still smell the vomit from the other night when I drank myself into oblivion.

It was light when I entered the room, but now it's covered with eerie shadows cast by the external floodlights outside my window. I wished I'd closed my blinds. But despite the light illuminating the dark night, all I can see is black. My eyes are open, staring at the bottom corner of my desk opposite me. I hadn't even noticed that's what my eyes were resting on until now. I am in a state of unconsciousness. My body is awake, but my mind is foggy like I've smoked too many bongs. My body is too heavy to lift off the ground, and until now I hadn't even realised I was on the ground.

I just want to be found. I want someone to notice I am cold and alone. I want someone to sneak into my room and find me here on the floor like I am every night and just know that I am not alright. I don't want to have to speak the words. I just want someone to know. I can't tell them what's going on because I can't even comprehend it myself.

I fear just sinking into the carpet like the Wicked Witch of the West melting into the floor. I beg for it. I want to dissolve into a liquid, unable to feel anymore. Thawing out of this frozen painful existence, vanishing into nothing. Evaporating into the essence of who I once was.

I don't want to be alone. I want to go home. But I fear the way I will be judged. I don't have a reason to not be okay. I've been trying to find one but none of them seem to fit. I just feel like everything is wrong but I can't quite put my finger on what it is. Is it my choice to go to law school that makes me so upset? Is it this location or campus that makes me so depressed? Is it my choice in friends that makes me wish I was dead? What is it about my life that makes me want so desperately to seek an end?

I'm stuck on a sinking ship. Please don't curse me for jumping overboard. I tried as hard as I could. Of that I am sure. But I'm sick of waiting for the tide to take my life. The sharks have been circling me for a while now. The end is near. I am not choosing to die, but I am terrified this awful disease will take my life. I crawl into bed and check my phone. "I'm dying," I whisper. It's just a matter of time before I enter the long eternal night. I begin my research on how to die.

What Is Wrong With Me?

Suicidal Barbie

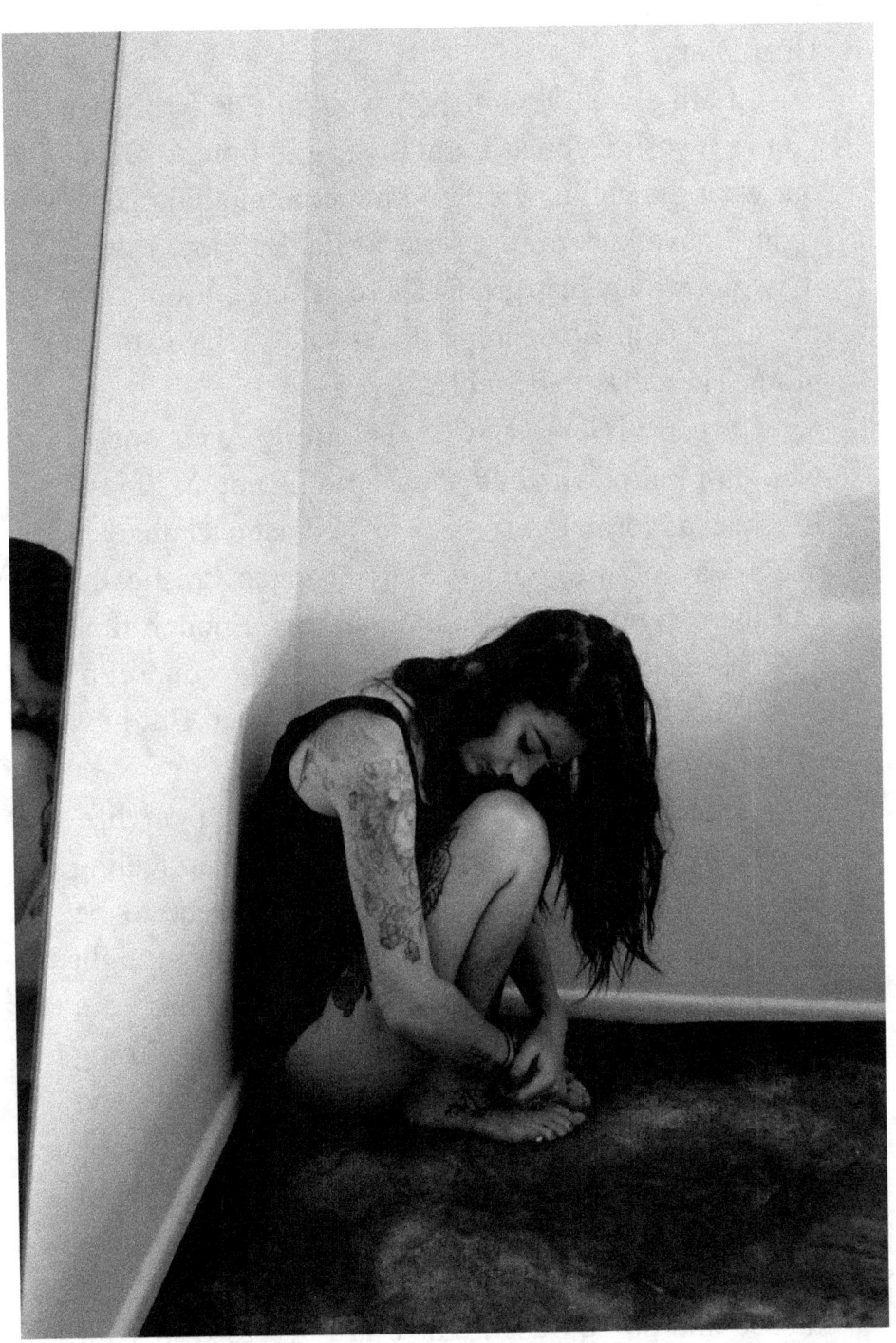

Dear Diary,

I am alive. Obviously. I wouldn't be writing in you if I wasn't. Since I am alive, it is time to figure out what the hell is wrong with me. Something is not right. I have known that for a while. But now I think it is more than just grief. There is more afoot than the mere pain of losing a loved one. I have to do more. There has to be more.

I can't *Google* what is wrong with me. I wouldn't know where to start. Grief is not an illness. It's just a normal response to a drastic change in one's way of life. My life has changed drastically. But there is nothing normal about this. Enough time has passed. I should have adjusted. My counsellor says I just have to learn to live without her. But how can I live without my mum?

I feel sad and down, but also high on life. Maybe it is just a coping mechanism to avoid feeling what I truly feel. I don't cry a lot. I seem to be beyond the point of crying. I've just skipped straight to the part where I stare off into space. I think I am living in a state of shock, denial and overwhelming numbness. I feel stressed, anxious, confused and exhausted all at the same time. I feel a lot of anger, grief, guilt, shame and resentment. I feel a lot of things. It all becomes a twisted ball of steel wool scrubbing away at my insides. The emotions are so intense and so confused that I struggle to deal with them. They give me headaches and keep me awake at night.

My brain is experiencing every natural disaster that humanity has ever experienced all at once. I feel the earthquakes shaking my foundations. I feel the fires burning in hell. I feel the hurricanes tear down everything I have built. The rain pours and the ice age freezes over everything else. My mind is seized by a bitter frost.

I smoke a pack of cigarettes a day. It is the only thing that brings me any relief. I don't know what else to do with myself. I breathe in the toxic smoke and exhale what little hope I have left. I feel tight in my chest and cough up phlegm. Maybe I am sick, maybe I am just sick of living like this. I must admit, my smoking is a cry for help. My tattoos are too. I am trying to change everything about me so people will see that something is wrong.

I cut my thighs in my room at night. I pick up the scissors or a knife and start to slide them along my skin. I am scared. I test myself to see how deep I am willing to go. I cut with anger and rage. I slice back and forth until I have a cross-stitched patch, swollen and sore across the top of my thighs. I squeeze the cuts until my quilt is beaded with blood. I no longer wear shorts. I try to hide my dirty little secret.

Sometimes I lift my shirt and cut the skin on

my stomach. I feel fat. I hate myself. The skin is sensitive there. It hurts just that little bit more. I can only bring myself to do it there when the self-hatred is so severe it outweighs the agony. Sometimes I like the pain. I like the risk. I like being able to be in control and feel something again. It releases years of built up tension.

It reminds me of being a young teenage girl, hiding in my room. I used to cut back then too. I did it to distract myself from the family war. I did it because I hated myself. I did it to punish myself for being such a stupid girl. I did it so that people would believe me when I said something was wrong. I did it to validate my pain. I did it to document the emotions I could not otherwise articulate.

Now that I smoke, I find myself burning my arms too. The cigarette burns are quite effective. They mark and scar with a lot less effort. I know people say I should put a rubber band on my wrist and flick it when I feel like this. But it's not the same. It isn't all about the pain. It is about what remains. It is the scar I yearn for. The physical representation of my pain. It is the lasting impact that I desire. It is a reminder of my emotional distress. It reminds me that I have been through a lot. It makes me feel like what I am going through is real and very significant. It reminds me that emotional pain is nothing compared to this numbness I feel every day. It helps bring me back to reality. It grounds me. Words just can't do justice to what I think and feel. There is no other way to capture the magnitude of my internal world.

Self-Harm Barbie

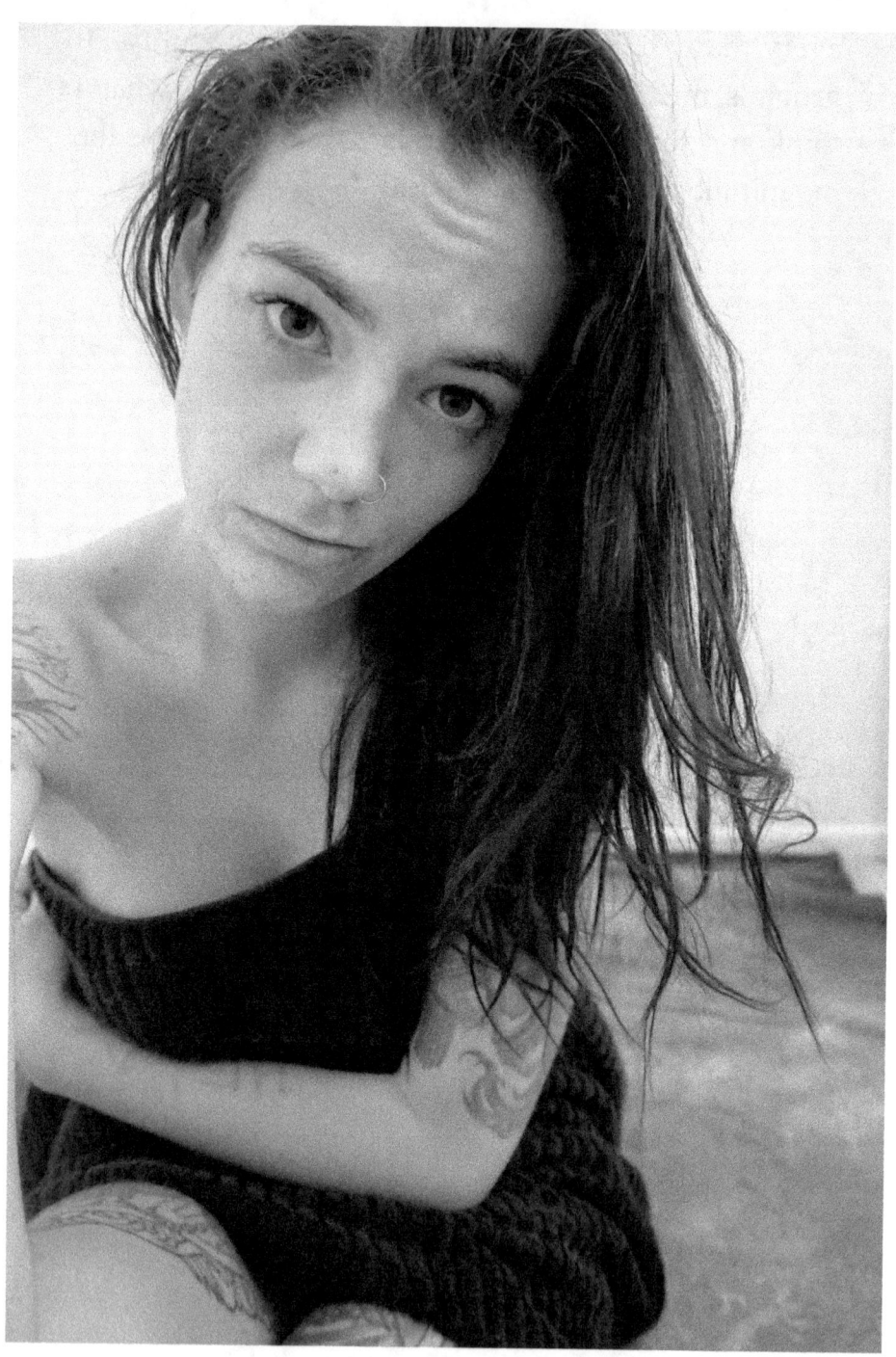

Dear Diary,

Today I feel completely exhausted, weak and drained. I feel like I am coming down with the flu, but I know I am not. Perhaps a more innocent or naïve version of me would have. I've been on edge for days; my heart is beating so fast it's bound to break down. Nowhere is safe, there is no rest for me. I am surrounded by a world I don't seem to fit into. A world I can't seem to get used to. A place that never feels like home. A fight that never ends and a war I just can't seem to win. It takes all of my strength just to be alive. To exist in such a state of fright. I have nowhere to run, nowhere to hide, I just suck it up and deal with it.

Is that not what I am expected to do?

I hate it when people tell me that putting my big girl pants on and going about life is what I have to do. It's even worse when they insinuate I am doing something else. I do that every second of every day! But it never gets easier. They might be able to suck up their problems like a vacuum cleaner and discard them in the trash, but I can't. My problem is me. Their troubles may pass, and in time they may be ok. But for me, it's the opposite. I suck it up each day until I manage to get to sleep at night knowing tomorrow will be more of the same. I pray each day for a better state of mind. But awake each morning to the same troubles every time.

I pray for a life that doesn't sting or a body that wants to stay in its own skin. A heart that does not overbeat and a mind that doesn't get frazzled and confused all of the time. I just want to rest, I just want to disappear, I just want to shrink, becoming so small it would be like I'm not alive at all.

I am about to pass out. Exhausted, I stare off into space. I don't even know what I am doing any more. Nervous tension has been buzzing through my body like ants in my pants, I can't sit down, so I pace around. I don't know what to do with myself, but I can't do anything either. Everything irritates me, even the air and the essence of my very existence feels like razor blades sliding across my skin.

Now I feel like I am going to drop dead. I am so out of it. I am so disoriented and exhausted it almost feels good. I am starting to become delusional, perhaps it is the bottle of red and three *Valiums* I just downed? I hope it knocks me out.

For now, I am alone with my thoughts. They are coming into the form of rhyme which happens from time to time. Perhaps I could be a poet? Or maybe a rapper?

    I yearn for rest, this feeling I detest.
    Each day is another test.
    Perhaps I'll fail them like all the rest.
    But there's not a minute's rest inside my head.

I fear I'll be left for dead with no more water left to tread.

I'll disappear onto the ocean bed.

A watery grave to mark my mistakes.

I'm fighting a war that has no end. My mind is a battlefield. A vast wasteland with a dark and ominous presence. The enemy is closing in. There are thousands of well trained and equipped soldiers marching straight towards me ready to attack. I look along my trenches and realise I am severely outnumbered. It's just me against my thoughts.

Emotions roll in like thunder bursting through the sky. They drop bombs from tanks shooting nasty feelings that blow up right in front of me. I want to run, but I am trapped in this hell hole entangled in barbed wire that fences me in. I have no choice but to fight as I can't run or hide. Believe me, I've tried. The enemy closes in, getting louder every time. They march towards me chanting their torment. They know no day or night, so the onslaught continues through to daylight, from dusk to dawn. In the dead of night, my mind is their hunting ground. They show no mercy. My mind is their oyster, and I am the pearl they wish to add to their crown. Defeat seems imminent as I search around, I can't seem to find a weapon. At least one that is big enough to conquer this beast that has emerged on this battlefield.

They send in the elite and I fear defeat.

I should retreat.

The future looks bleak.

The dirt turns to mud beneath my feet, and I slip and fall down.

I desperately want a shower or a place to drown.

That's where I go when I need to disappear for a moment or two.

I feel detached from my body. I am caged in my own skin. There is simply no escape!

Each day is a new opportunity they say, but I know better now. Each day a new beast is trying to tear me down. They show no remorse. I isolate myself from the world because I can't bear to be around myself so why would anyone else?

I don't feel like myself. I'd hate for them to see me like this, to judge me like this. This person I don't want to be, but I don't have a choice.

Sometimes I zone out, and I don't know what happens in that period of time that is blocked out. I only realise I've been gone when I return to reality and wish I could go back to where I was. I get annoyed, angry and mad when I am distracted from my thoughts. People encourage me to get out of my head, to bring me back down to reality to make me engage with the world. But what they can't comprehend is that I'm fighting a war inside my head! Pull my attention away from the battlefield and all of a sudden I am slaughtered by the enemy. Distract me for a moment and blood will be shed. I am under siege 24/7. An automatic weapon fires each and every second, a bullet penetrates my skin. I want to live in the world, but I can't do both. Not when it's this severe, and the enemy won't back down. I try to negotiate a ceasefire, but depression won't hear me out. Sometimes I can when the war isn't as grim. But bullets fly, shrapnel is propelled through the air, and I fear I may be left for dead. 'Leave no man behind' doesn't really apply in a war of the mind.

I want to retreat, I want to surrender, but that's not an option when your life is on the line, and the enemy won't back down. When people ask why I would want to take my own life I simply reply with a frown, "I'm ending the war I've been losing for a while now, I see no other way out."

I don't expect them to wrap their head around a suicide attempt. I know that they can't see inside my head or comprehend why I would rather be dead. They think my fight is a lie because it's invisible to them. If they looked hard enough, they might just find they were mistaken and just ignored the signs. My messy room, the dishes in a pile, a replica of the leaning tower of stale old pizzas. They call me lazy and order me to clean it up. In their mind, I am just a massive let down.

I marvel at how well I can multitask. Fighting a war inside my head while living a life I don't want to live amidst the mess that seems to surround me. I don't choose to back down or admit defeat. But I can't keep fighting two battles at once and stay up on my feet. The battle to stay alive isn't won trying to keep a job, manage finances, be sociable or hanging my washing out. Dealing with the demons in my head – or the emotions that surge through my body like an electric shock – is a full-time job in itself.

Depression wraps its big monstrous arms around me and puts me in a headlock. It follows me around constantly attacking me and knocking me down to the ground. It attacks me whenever I let my guard down. My stomach is tied in knots as I am bound by the troubles I can't run from. My journey is profound, but I am yet to be found by the ones I love. Maybe when I'm six feet underground, they might start to see that I wasn't messing around.

I haven't won every battle and maybe I never will, but losing a few doesn't mean I'm giving up entirely. Some days I am just too outnumbered. Sometimes I have to give up on life just to conquer the battle of the day in my mind. It's like I'm somewhere inside fighting for control of myself, hating the person I have temporarily become but can't shake her off as she clings to me like a monkey hitching a ride on my back!

Soldier Barbie

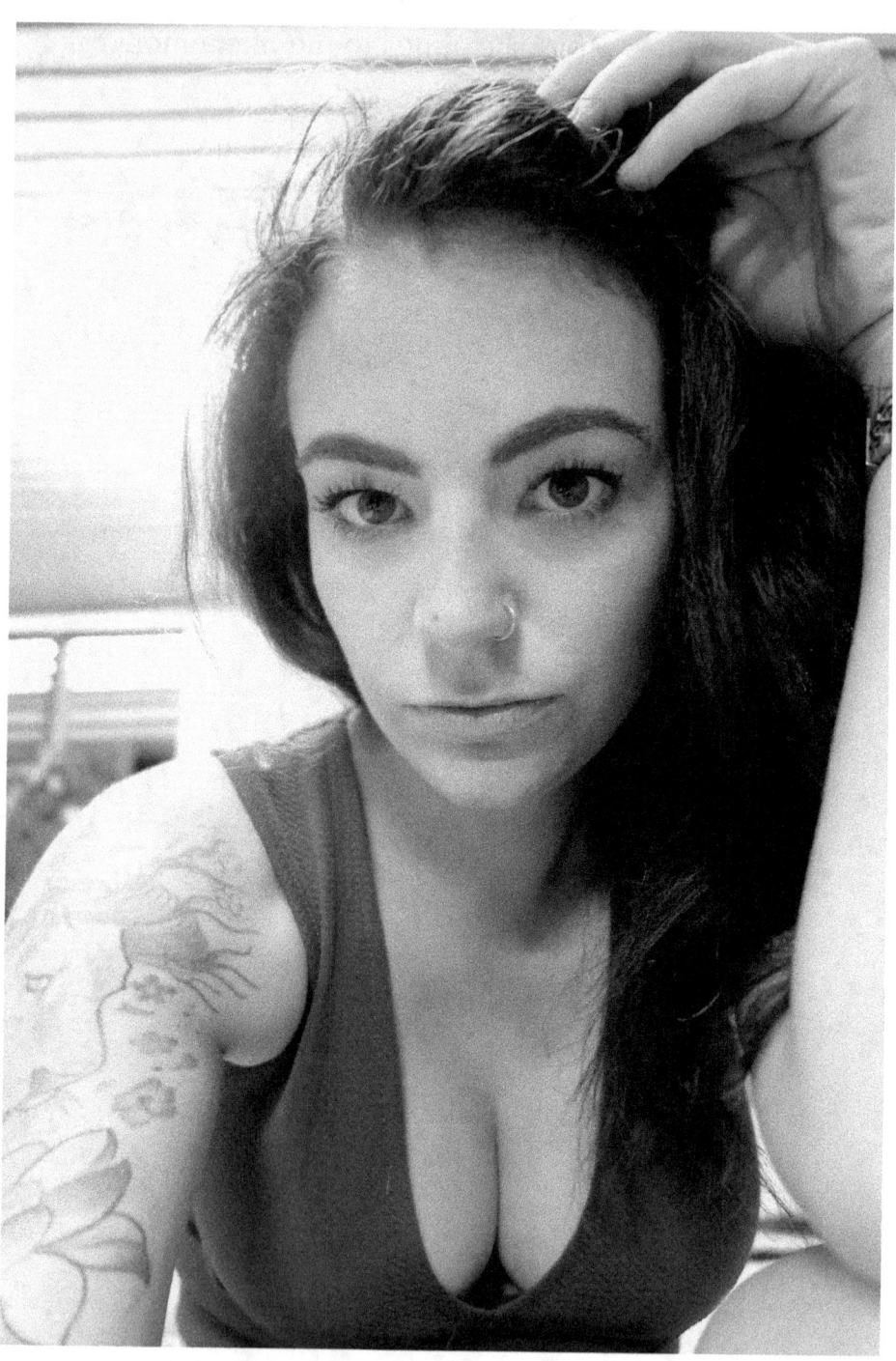

Dear Diary,

Fear is a funny thing. Sitting on my swing today a big snake slithered right up to me. Before I consciously knew what I was doing, I grabbed my dog who wanted to greet this unfamiliar creature and made a run for it. Just minutes before I had been sitting in the sun. Telling the universe, I was done and asking it to please put me out of my misery. I wasn't sad. I was content with my decision. I confirm it every day. Perhaps an opportunity presented itself, but before I knew it, I had saved myself.

It's always the way. Whether it be vomiting up a belly of pills or clawing your way to the surface choking on water. Something strange happens when you decide to die. Subconsciously your body is programmed to survive. That is our primary instinct and no matter how hard we try to give up, we can't help but fight. But that doesn't mean we are alright.

When people ask me if I am okay, I ask them how they define the word? Because each day I am okay and not, all at the same time. My bar for being alright is set so low. I've been living like this for so long, it's my version of normal. It's the baseline at which I live my life. Maybe if people knew what it was like for me to be always drowning with my head at the tip of the surface. Never asking for help until I am fully submerged. But by then, it's too late. No one can hear my screams from under the water. So even though I may be bobbing like a cork on the surface, that doesn't mean I don't always need saving. I want to save myself, and I don't really have any other choice. But I fight so many battles that even if I've won most of them, one victory alone is still not worth this life.

I am alright. I just wish more people understood my life. Maybe then I wouldn't feel like the only thing I'm fighting for is to prove that what I fight against is real. Maybe it will feel like all this effort was for something. I'm not sure what I find more unbelievable: how many times I can muster my last bit of hope to reach out just one more time, or how much more it hurts each time I am rejected? Maybe it's how surprised I seem to feel each time another dead end or roadblock appears when I do reach out for help. Whether it be another uncooperative, invalidating, patronising medical professional, a disheartening conversation about how I can't be helped – leaving me feeling completely helpless – or stigma fuelled advice from professionals sworn to help the unwell.

I expect it from my friends and family or the general public. I know my cries for help are bound to fall on deaf ears. No one wants to hear someone else's problems. They preach about reaching out, but reaching out for me has never been a problem. Finding someone who is willing to listen and really hear me speak is the first – almost unattainable – hurdle. It's a miracle if they are qualified or have any remote knowledge on what to do.

They might turn a blind eye to our "cries for help" when it affects them or is noticeably destructive. But someone only cries for help when they believe help is available. I am living proof that no matter how hard you try, no matter how many people you reach out to, there just isn't enough help available. Whether it be cost issues, availability issues, a lack of qualified professionals at your disposal or a ridiculous secretive government system that is designed to "help" us but all it seems to do is make the difficult commitment to getting better seem like a figment of my childish imagination. Their claims are so vastly different from the reality that it took me many years to lose the naïve hope that this world is worth living in.

Having my hopes and dreams of a life I might actually enjoy living defeated by the only people who can help me find a way to live in this world is what drives me towards suicide. I decided many years ago that I couldn't go on living like this and ever since then there is only one thing I do and think of every second of every day and that is how can I find a way to live and have even the tiniest bit of life quality?

So far I have been unsuccessful in my quest.

When is it okay to say you have had enough? When does a parent give up hope that their missing child will return home alive? How long am I expected to be the walking dead before I can finally be laid to rest?

Suicidal Barbie

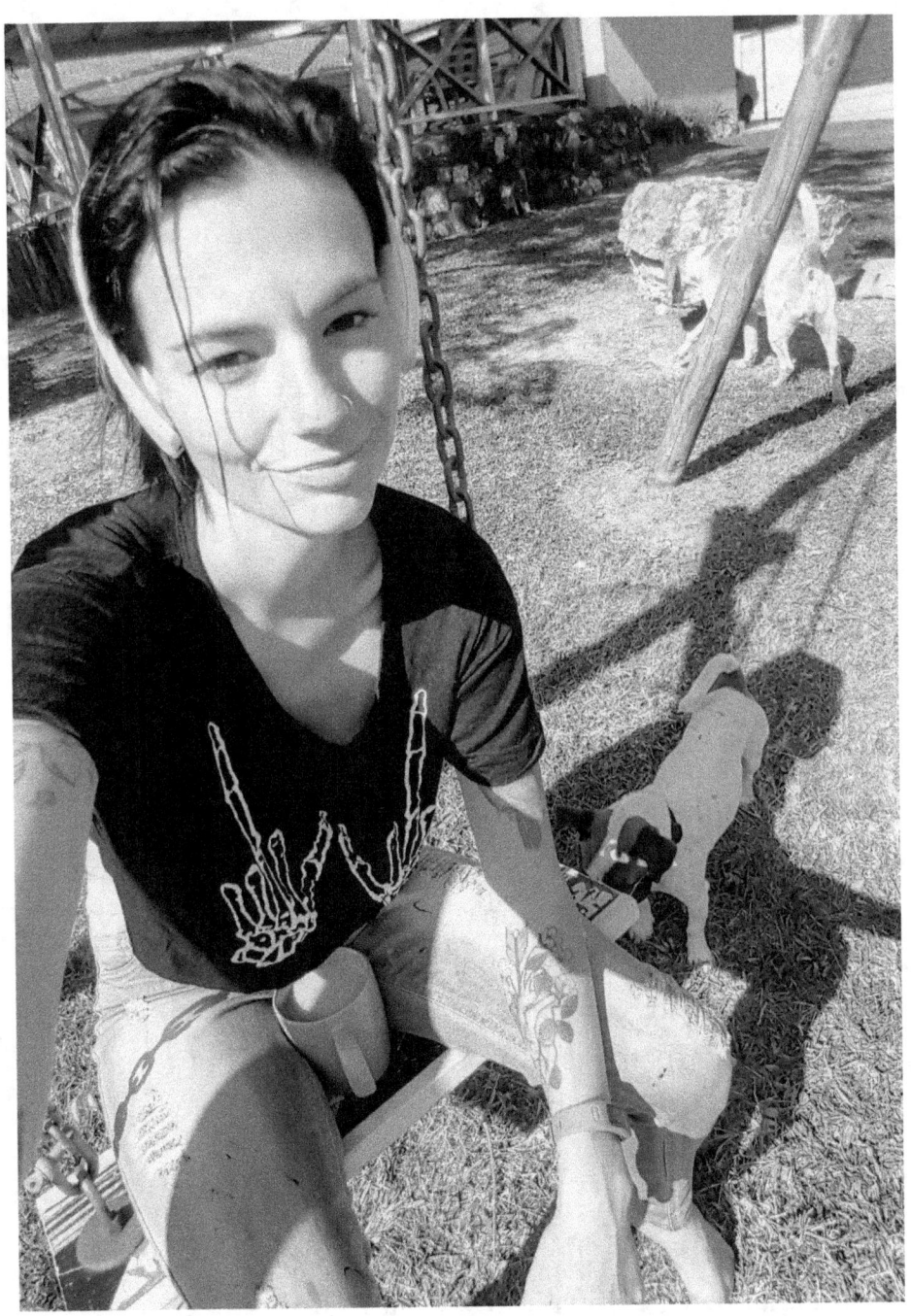

Dear Diary,

Things in my mind are broken, and things in my life are fucked! (For lack of a better word.) Home doesn't feel like home. But neither does anywhere else. Nowhere feels safe. If I'm being honest, it never did. I am consumed by worry, fear and anxiety. I am the thought police, constantly trying to catch the thoughts that creep so sneakily into my mind, trying to sabotage my happiness. The other symptoms come in waves. They crash over my body with such sudden force that sometimes they knock me down. Or they bring me up in a state of turmoil where I don't know which way is down or which is up; I couldn't figure it out if my own life depended on it!

I am trapped in the whitewash of life and mental illness. I am halfway between shore and the deeper depths of the endless ocean. The day is sunny and bright, but it couldn't be further from the way I feel. The pain is unbearable as I forced myself to drag my body around in this world. It used to be something that wasn't a problem for me, but I knew now that it really had been eating away at me for years.

Deep down inside I felt like an empty shell of what I used to be before the depression set in. When this happens, I don't know what to do. I never really do. Does anybody?

I have learnt a lot and try with all my might to find the shallows of life to bring just enough balance to survive. But I don't just want to survive. I want to thrive. It seems like a luxury I can't seem to grasp. My heart races, I feel so strange. Crippling anxiety is trying to tear me down. Worry is my constant companion, and rightly so, life is unfair. People and places and things seem to always end in despair. I feel unreal, surreal alone but never left alone. I live in constant paradoxes.

Fear is my enemy, but the only friend I have. I hope others will never know the torment I feel on this day or the one before that. Why is this happening to me? I am just a simple girl, or at least I was before things changed, and life became complex. Life suddenly filled with stress as happiness left. I entered the 'worry world'. A place where I can't sleep for days or weeks or months.

Sometimes I want to die for no reason at all. Except maybe the fact that the life I live is hard. Life is hard, too hard. It is incredibly difficult and hard to bear at times. Every day in fact. But I fight on. For what? I'm not even sure anymore.

I am trapped in my mind, there's no escape. No safe place. There is nowhere I can rest my head to get some shut-eye. There is nowhere I can go to shut off the lights just for a moment in time. So I escape to the only places I know. I escape even further into my head. I escape beyond my conscious mind; I travel deeper than the troubles I find. I escape to a world I create deep inside this vast endless space. I disassociate to a better place, a show I direct. It's an escape from the burdens of life I find so hard to digest.

I feel broken down, my body aches, my head hurts from these persistent migraines. My heart has no time to bleed from past mistakes. I deal with what I have to, one step at a time. I use all my therapy training to get through each day. To survive in this life that constantly tries to break me. I don't know which way is up. Everything around me is constantly changing. I struggle to find direction in a life so full of turmoil. Because I don't know where to go. There's no escape for me. Every path I take I just seem to stumble further down the rabbit hole.

I fight hard to maintain contact with the ones I know, yet the fear of being hurt cripples me as I feel my chest cave in.

"Do I look sick? Do I look hopeless? Do I hide it all well?" I ask myself. I don't think so. I think acne is a tell-tale sign of my distress. I hate that my face looks like I have caught the plague as volcanic pimples erupt all over the place. I don't know whether it's the hormones or the amount of time I spend with my head in my hands. Is stress a bacteria?

I know that others can't see my headaches, but they always hear me mentioning them. Ever heard of a stress headache? Probably not. They have heard of chronic fatigue and insomnia or the terrible consequences of sleep deprivation. But no one talks about how I am tired all the time.

I don't understand why people always, always, ALWAYS feel a need to blame me for all these symptoms. I can't be fatigued because I am sick, I just want to be fatigued. I can't be tired because I am worn out and exhausted, I am just lazy. It's like once your symptoms get linked to mental illness, then others think they are off the hook. It's like a free pass for them to skip offering support, emotionally or physically. It's like a card that allows them to discredit me and disregard any physical complaint I may have. It's like saying to someone with cervical cancer, "Oh get over it, it just means it will slightly inconvenience your sex life nothing else." Or saying to someone with breast cancer, "Meh, breast cancer is super common these days, you'll be alright". Wouldn't it sound ridiculous if we switched the word depression or anxiety with cancer? Imagine what that would sound like if people said to them what they say to me?

At the end of the day, everything stays the same. No one understands why I struggle. How, I ask, can anyone survive in a world where chaos and hate overtake? Every bit of happiness is sucked out or tries to escape. The laughter and smiles I manage to muster never seem to last because I am haunted by memories of my past and taunted by the grim reality of battling yet another day.

These are the days of my life, in a soap opera where I am the star of the show. I feel like my life is a less glamorous version of *The Bold and the Beautiful*. I no longer scream for help because like the children I cared for in orphanages all over the world, I know no one will hear. People don't cry for help when it isn't there.

My demons torment me daily, breaking the woman who was once very strong. A woman who is still very strong but wary of this daily contest. I see no end in sight for some parts of this journey. I will surely still suffer for years to come. But yet I fight on. Why? I am stronger than the people who hurt me and the sickness that threatens to kill me. I can guarantee that!

Defective Barbie

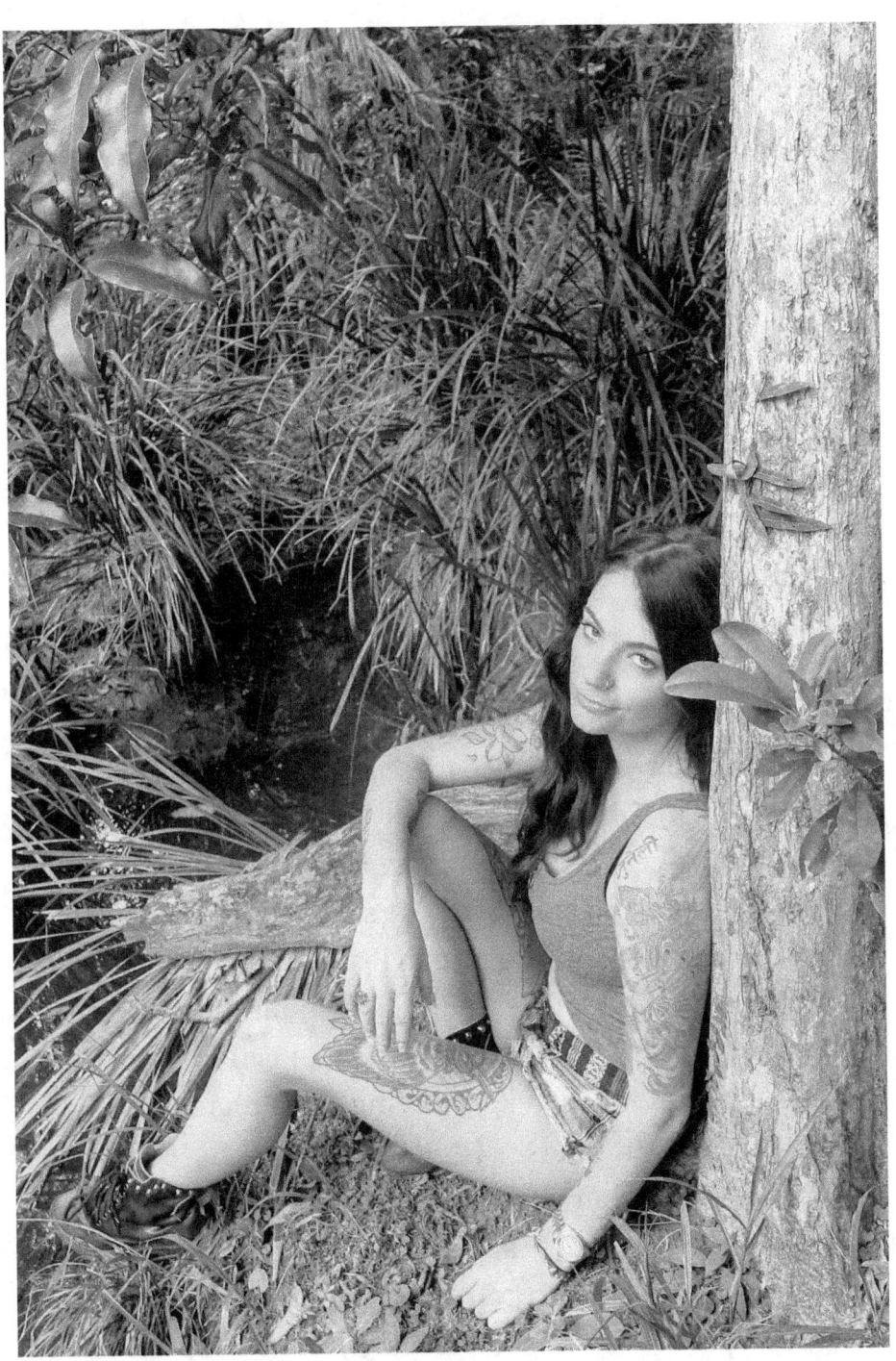

Dear Diary,

After a terrible day of severe depression I walked into my therapist's office with a heavy heart and slumped into the couch. I didn't have to look around the room to get my bearings. I have been here more times than I can count. I am surprised at how long she has stuck around. She is my seventh therapist I have had over the years. I go for a while and then just get too depressed to attend appointments anymore. I avoid their calls to check in and when they stop and I am ready to talk again, I feel too embarrassed to reach out. So I go without until things get so bad I need to see someone. I go to the GP to get a referral to a new one and then book the next available appointment. Usually next available for new clients means three to six months for anyone worth seeing. They also charge an arm and a leg even with the *Medicare* rebate. I still have to fork out hundreds of dollars I never have. That just creates another reason I miss appointments. Maybe that's why they book them so far in advance? So people have a chance to save up? I certainly don't have enough funds to keep seeing them regularly.

Then of course I move state and location prevents me from seeing a familiar face. I have had my fair share of first appointments. The ones where you have an hour to tell your whole life story and open up old wounds before they tell you time is up and ask you to book an appointment two weeks from now. Most of the time in therapy I have spent is just allowing my therapist to learn my story. I never seem to get to the helpful part.

"How are you today?" she asked me, her voice gentle as if breaking a fragile eggshell. I let out an exasperated sigh, shutting my eyes to try and forget everything for just a moment or two. My therapist interrupted my thoughts with one of her own; "Do you want to tell me what happened that made your day so bad?"

I shook my head violently from side to side, but eventually relented after being cajoled by the gentle voice of my therapist who had been treating me for some time now.

I was reminded to look back at how far I have come. I've realised it's easy to feel like you are not making any progress when everything around you still looks the same. When your life is still a mess, you still feel crap, and it doesn't seem like you have even made an inch of progress, I try to remind myself that recovery is a journey, not a destination. You can't transport yourself there with a simple thought.

Survival is a natural human instinct but escaping that deserted island is a choice. It requires skills, determination and education. While I am still lost at sea surrounded by water-soaked horizons, I sometimes forget that I am slowly developing my sea legs. I am in uncharted territory that I am gradually beginning to map.

First I must find out where I am, then which direction I need to head in and how to get there before I can make any progress at all. I am thankful that I now know what I am dealing with and for the medical team I have around me to help me do just that.

I decided to spend an hour going over the positive things that had happened to me. It was motivation to get back on track with my life.

Cartographer Barbie

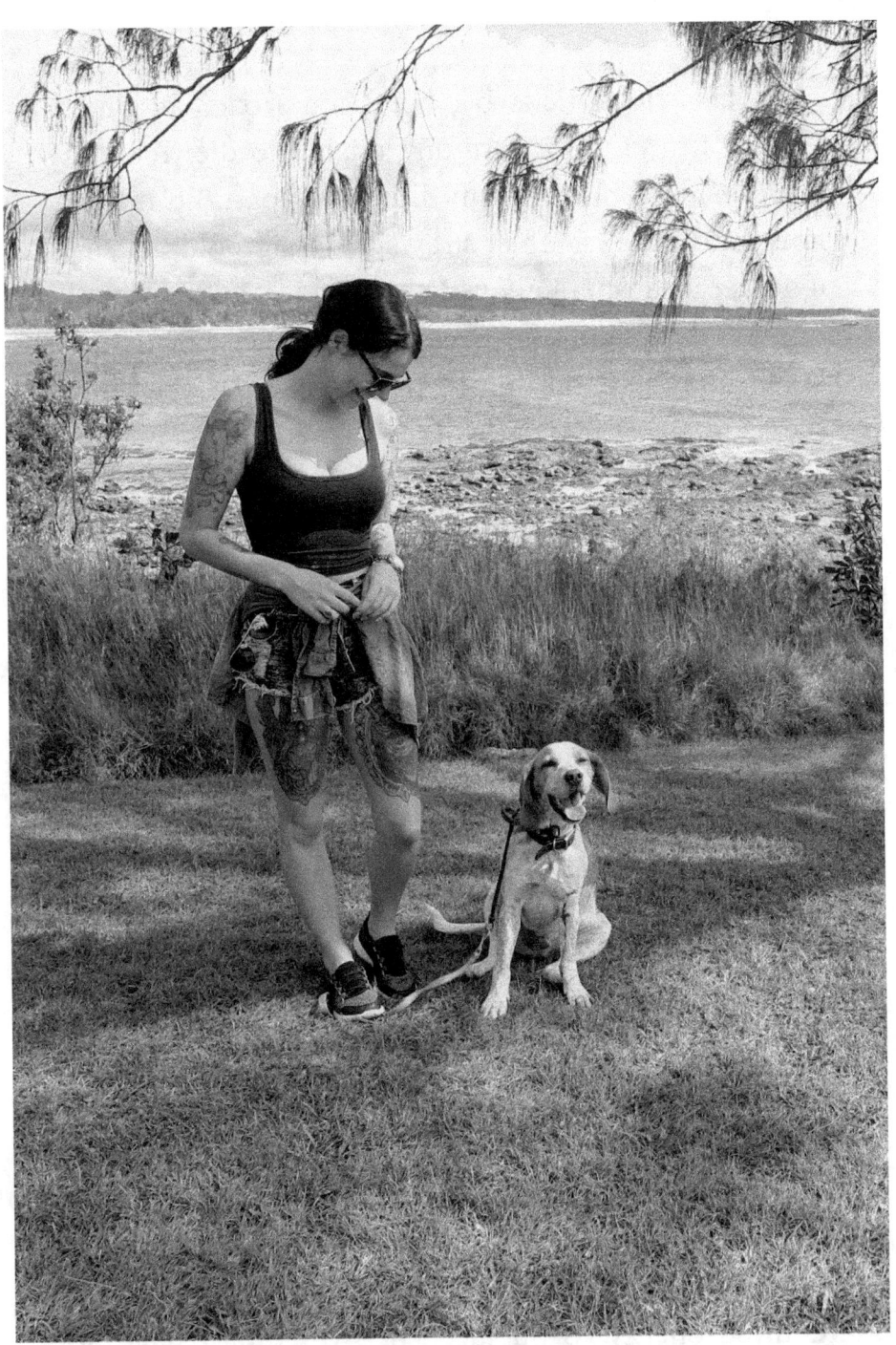

Dear Diary,

The clock ticks by, but I am frozen in time. Unable to move forward and unable to die. I watch my dreams drift by as my life falls apart, no matter how hard I try. I grab at straws trying to hold my shit together as desperately as I can to ride out this storm. The winds are getting stronger, the waves are getting taller, and I am starting to lose sight of it all. Time seems to pass too quickly. I try to meditate as I sit on my bed and listen to the rain outside. My mind keeps drifting onto the topic of accommodation. I try to bring my awareness back to the bed I sit on and to be grateful that I have a place to sleep tonight. No matter the shitty situation I intend to make lemonade out of a bunch of rotten lemons.

I take a deep breath and think of the three beautiful paintings I dropped off on consignment today. My art is now displayed in wonderful venues. I remind myself that it is tough moments like these that might have been incredibly hard to endure, but have given me opportunities like this. It has made my art better and more thought-provoking. It engages people on a deeper level than the perfect little animals I drew ever did.

At the beginning of today, I'd felt like it was a shame none of that mattered. I couldn't even enjoy those moments, those big achievements because they required energy to pursue. Energy I didn't have at my disposal. I was spent and ready for bed. But despite having very difficult discussions all day, my day was turned around by a very amazing conversation with an equally amazing woman. I am touched, my heart beats brighter tonight after our chance encounter. She left me speechless, a feat not many achieve! She definitely changed the tone of my day from hopelessness and desperation to optimism and endless possibilities. I am incredibly grateful for that. She reminded me by believing in what I am trying to do that it is something incredibly special and her faith in my eventual success made me regain mine.

I am left with a sweet question in my mind: Do I live it safe? Or do I take a chance on the unknown? Safe hasn't gotten me very far yet. In fact, safe has nearly always let me down. There's room for disappointment in the realm of safety. If I take a chance and it could very much fail, the odds really aren't that different to playing it safe.

Hope comes from the strangest of places sometimes. I am terrified of the good and bad possibilities of the future. But I now have hope again. Of a brighter future. As I embrace two-and-a-half hours of dance tonight, I am in my element! I can forget the troubles of the day. Troubles that have been turned into opportunities with a hint of light instead of dark high walls I can't quite see over. I ask myself the very pressing question as I dance across the floor. Why not? Fears that held me back from dancing for years. Fear of failure that kept me from this beautiful happy place I escaped to. When I ask myself the question now, and my only answer is fear, do I take this challenge and opportunity in the same way I dance? In facing that fear, I opened myself up to the amazing possibilities I now enjoy. I was terrified of dancing, I deprived myself of something I now love so much because I was scared.

Taking a dance class is a little less scary than moving to the other side of the country. Melbourne is a long way from home and a long way from anyone I know. Is that threatening or appealing? I am not too sure. Being able to reinvent myself would be nice. I would like to disappear and have some time to heal. In a way, it's kind of a fuck you to everyone over here who didn't believe in me. It would be nice to leave and then return one day as everything they told me I wasn't. Maybe I really should just leave and give them a taste of what life would be like without me. I can't help but wonder if my urge to run away is clouding my judgement?

When I asked for advice on the matter tonight, my wise dance instructor said to me, "There are three things you need to consider when asking for advice and you should only take on board someone's advice if they fit all three. Do they know you well?

Have they lived in your shoes, struggled with the things you have, faced similar obstacles? And have they been where you want to go? That resonated with me tonight. If I am honest ... then no one I know fits that criteria except maybe a special lady I met today. My goals and aspirations are in relatively uncharted territory. No one I know would ever dream of doing the things I know I will achieve in my life. No one truly knows me better than I know myself. I have a hard time convincing anyone else of that though. I ask myself who I am. What do I want? I know what I want. Who I am is a little more difficult to figure out. Do we ever truly know?

Maybe this is just going to be another massive mistake. I must acknowledge those mistakes that have made me into the person I am today. All mistakes began as opportunities, even if they didn't work out. It really is what you make the most of. Regardless of what I choose to do, there's the potential for it to be another mistake or the best decision of my life. Either way, it's my choice, and I have to make sure not to let others influence it. At the end of the day, I am the one that has to live with the consequences.

Hopeful Barbie

Who knew that all this time, there was a drowning girl hiding behind that smile.

Bipolar Barbie

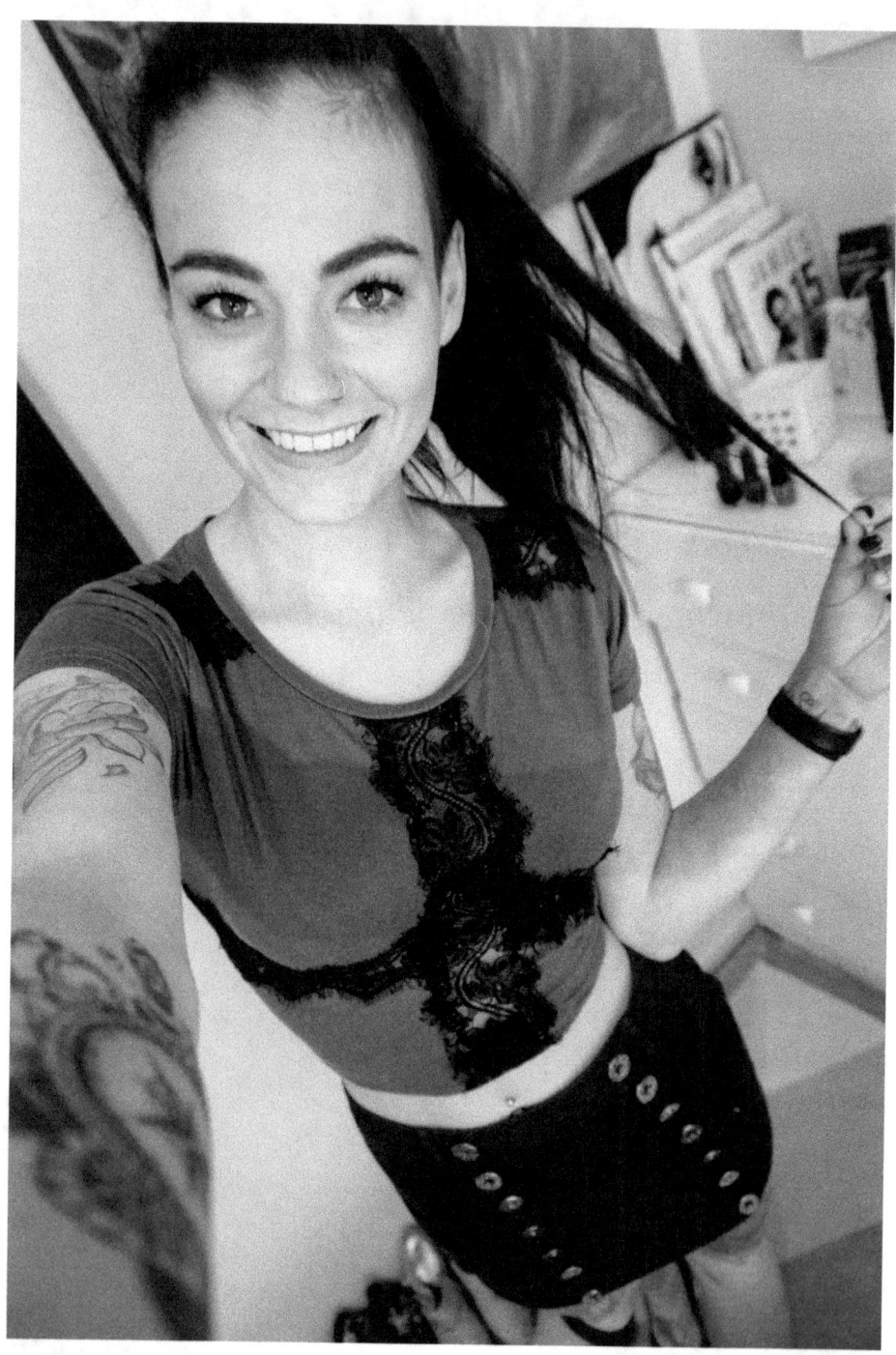

Dear Diary,

It's a strange thing to watch your mental health deteriorate. At first you notice the instability, like you are balancing on the edge of a cliff. A sly glance, an inappropriate, insensitive comment can tip you over the edge at any moment. It's like always dancing on the lip of your breaking point. Everything else fades away. The world becomes dark and you are staring down the rabbit hole. You suddenly feel five inches tall and too small to be safe in such a dark place. You are too afraid to do anything because everything cuts like a knife, but you are also beyond feeling pain. Pain is your new normal. Torment is now your way of life. Torture is what you have to look forward to every day when you wake up. Sleeping provides relief, but the double-edged sword is on the other side of sleep when you wake up. A fresh start. The devil resets the time loop and you live your worst nightmares all over again.

It's like witnessing the suffering of a loved one as they knock on death's door. But worse, because that someone is you. It is hard to watch yourself shrink further and further within yourself. To watch your enthusiasm and motivation dissipate. Your energy levels drop to catastrophic lows. Fatigue becomes you and exhaustion consumes you. Your body grows so incredibly heavy, and you begin to sink within your own skin. Tears well up in your eyes and you don't even know why. This overwhelming sense of loss and loneliness sweeps over you. You stop living and just seem to exist in a situation, and you have no idea how you ended up here. You see no way out. It's like falling down a big hole and hitting your head, waking up and realising you can no longer see daylight.

Time and time again you find yourself pondering your own existence. You realise you don't value your own life anymore. Nothing seems to matter. Nothing piques your interest, and you have no apparent feelings towards anything. Everything seems like too much effort, even breathing is a burden. You have been working so hard for so long to overcome everything you are forced to face. You are tired and worn out. Your aspirations lay in the mud around you as you collapse to the ground knowing that dreams are for princesses in fairy tales, of which you are not. How can you delude yourself into thinking you could be something when you can't even find a stable place to sleep or enough food to eat? What you ask for is not much, but someone thinks it's too much. How else would you be in this situation in life?

Year after year you begin to wonder what it was you did so wrong to warrant this type of eternal punishment? Surely I have done my time? If not a thousand times over. It seems so inhumane.

There's a cure they preach, you just have to try. Try to be happy, try to smile, try to be everything you are not. Just hide your pain and swallow your guilt. I tried, but I choked on it.

Everyone has their own conflicting ways of dealing with it and I have tried them all, but unlike them, I see no success. I do everything right; I seek help, go to therapy, take medication and live a "happy" lifestyle. I think positive thoughts and research anything and everything that could ease my state of mind. I find things that temporarily relieve my symptoms but the gains are so small and far apart they barely seem to count.

All I want is for someone to understand and be there for me when I need it most. But I am too scared to ask, not wanting to be a burden or risk being rejected like I have many times before. Anything anyone says in this vulnerable time, in my darkest hour of need seems to make me feel less loved than before I spoke. I am labelled as a burden or attention seeking so I put on a fake smile because I don't want to cause concern. Torn between hitting the panic button and waiting for the storm to pass. They say it will, but it might not. And if this is really the lowest of my lows maybe I don't want anyone to know. Secretly praying to find the courage to end my suffering with finality.

I wasn't always this defeated. I thought I found a lifeboat. I seemed stable for a while. I fought for my life and tried to hold on. When I yelled for help I screamed with laughter to hide my own guilt.

Why ask for help if it will do no good? Why reach out for the thousandth time to feel even more helpless than before? I wouldn't mind if my cries for help fell on deaf ears and in a way they do; how could anyone not know? Being stigmatised by family and loved ones hurt the most. They say they will miss me if I die. But ask yourself this, where were you in my life? Why was it I chose to take my own life if you all cared so much? Where were you all those days I contemplated suicide? Where are you tonight?

Funny how when you're dead people start listening …

Suicidal Barbie

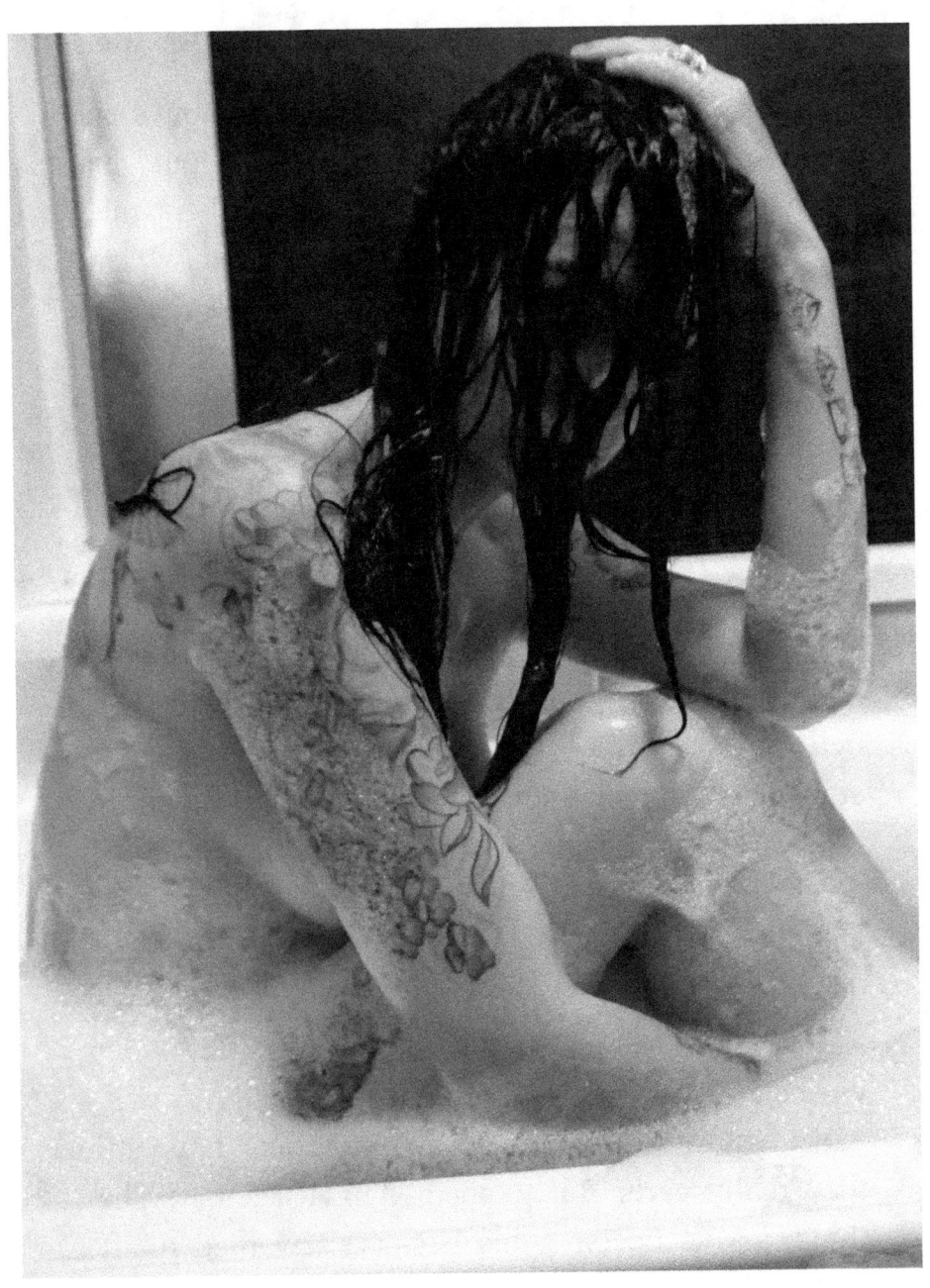

Dear Diary,

I've become so numb over the years, but I can still feel their hurtful stares. I didn't realise that I had become numb to the world until after it happened. My face was frozen in a permanent scowl, my eyebrows furrowed as if they were constantly in pain, and my eyes narrowed so much that I could barely see anything around me. Covered by an oversized hoodie and dark sunglasses, nobody ever really saw my features. Nobody knew who or what I was anymore; not even myself.

I can feel the way they judge me, and each word they speak hurts like knives being thrown at me. Their only goal is to shoot me down. They believe what I face isn't real, so they discredit my story every chance they get, to break down this illusion they think I'm hiding behind. But the joke's on them. Because it's not an illusion. It's very real, and their attempts to tear down my "excuse" just adds to the pain.

I'm so tired and so aware of what's really going on inside my mind. It highlights the vastly growing gap of how little others really know and how little they really care. But to them, I'm just a liar. They think I have become this because I wanted to. It's like all I ever wanted to do is be a fuck up. But the truth is I'm just more like me and a hell of a lot less like them. I understand how terrifying that must be for them. To lose someone you once knew. But I'm losing myself too.

I don't understand how they can't see I'm being smothered by something they won't even acknowledge exists. I'm suffocating in a bubble you claim to see right through; it's invisible to you. To you, I've lost control. But in reality I am terrified of losing control. Everything you thought I would be has fallen apart. But I've forgotten who I wanted to be. I am drowning, you just don't know.

So please don't you dare judge me for being sick. Don't you dare speak a word to me because everything that comes out of your mouth just turns to ash the minute you say it. I don't expect you to say the right thing. But you're more than willing to say the wrong thing. I'm just a disgrace to you. A waste of space. Every word you speak makes me feel like everything I have tried so hard not to be.

It is always the same. I talk and they stare with their judging eyes and their twitching lips. It is as if they can see right through me as if my clothes were transparent. Or so they think. It isn't that I don't want to be seen; it's just that I wanted for them to see me for who I really am – not what they think of me when they see a mentally ill tattooed person.

They can't see the things that tie me down or the cement boots cast upon my legs. I just sink below their gaze like the sun hiding beyond the horizon. They have faith that I will rise again tomorrow. But they have no idea how close I am to taking my final breath.

Alone Barbie

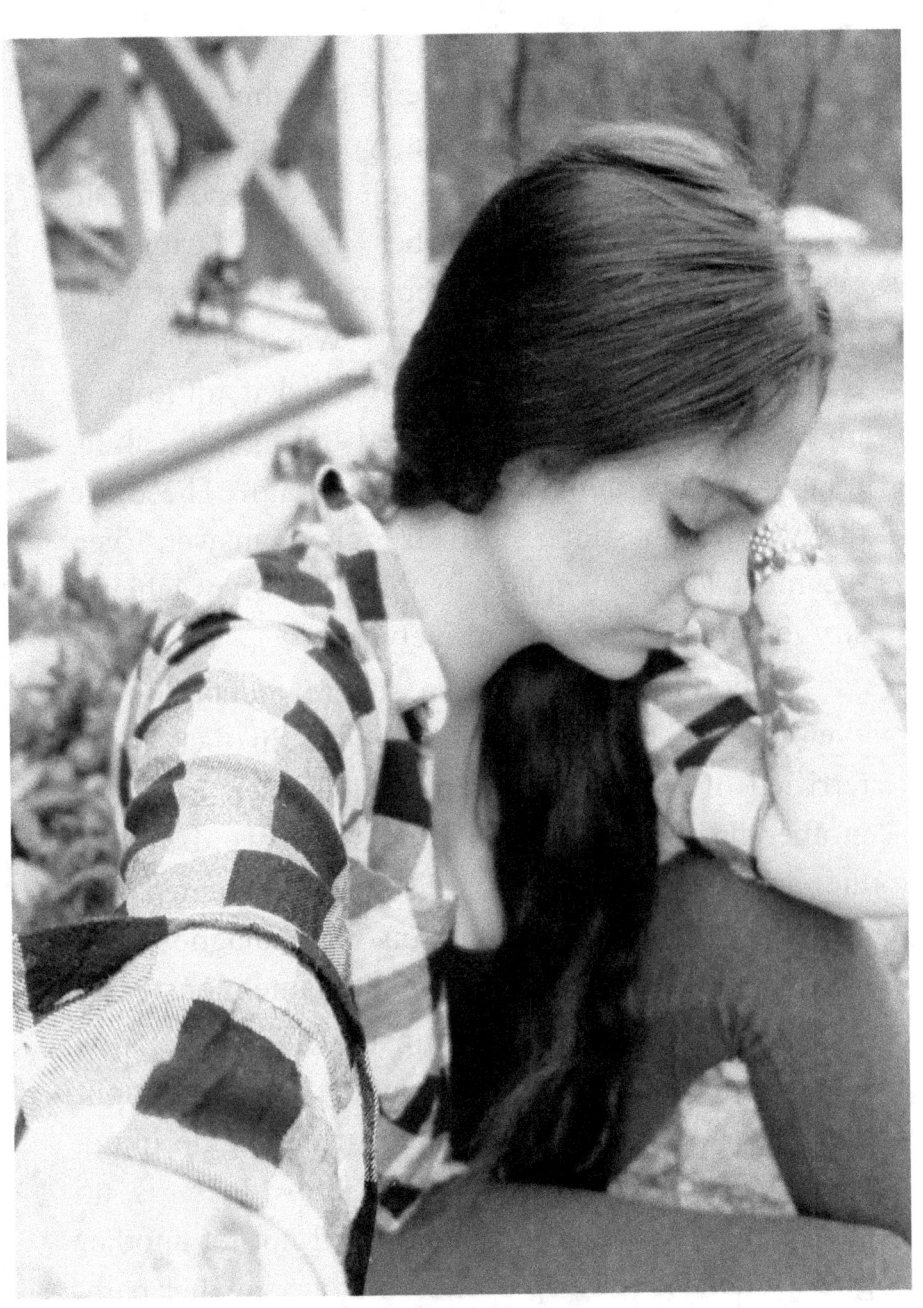

Dear Diary,

Looking back now it seems that this wasn't the first time I had experienced a type of depression. It just seemed like I used to handle it a lot better. Did the trauma of that September in 2012 trigger a sleeping dragon? Was my Bipolar Disorder just lying dormant waiting to be exposed? Was it inevitable? Could I have prevented it or avoided it infiltrating my life if I had not experienced this heartbreaking tragedy? Can trauma rewire your brain? These are the types of questions I still struggle to answer. Even the most learned experts in the field of psychiatry struggle to answer it definitively.

I don't think having a severe mental illness ever crossed my mind. Not at first. In fact I was terrified of ever getting Bipolar Disorder. My birth mother has severe mental illness and we'd always thought she had bipolar disorder. I blamed her erratic, abusive behaviour on that diagnosis. It terrifies me that I could become the same monster.

I am faced with discrimination and expectation that compels me to share my journey so others might not have to feel so alone. I wear my struggle like a badge of honour so that others know there is no shame in what we go through. I will not let another girl cry herself to sleep because no one saw her pain. I will not let another little girl's problems be cast aside or shrugged off as insignificant because I know how it feels. I know how natural it is to come to the conclusion that if my problems are insignificant, so am I. If I am insignificant, then I don't deserve to be alive. I won't let another child contemplate their life because someone made them feel unworthy for having a story to tell.

It makes me mad that there are other people who have to deal with the rejection I felt. Despite everything I've been through, I have accepted I'm here for a greater purpose and while that idea sounds absurd in itself, that's what keeps me going. It allows me to see the light through a dark and cloudy storm. It allows me to find a silver lining in even the worst of situations.

I know what it's like to fight this battle and feel alone. I think the alone part is the worst of it all. We are all here for a reason. Even my crappy marriage and divorce; I've managed to see a reason for that. I know my reason in his life was to get him to Melbourne to become the best chef around. I succeeded in that. Maybe I am yet to figure out what he did for me, but it taught me some things I may have never otherwise learnt. As many other people have come into my life to teach me valuable lessons.

Suffering can be temporary or last a lifetime if you let it. Holding on to all of that anger, regret, disappointment and resentment prolongs your suffering. Just because something should not have happened doesn't mean you have to let it affect the rest of your life. Everything is meant to be. That's the faith I believe in. The faith that keeps me navigating the treacherous waters of life. Even with broken sails.

Lonely Barbie

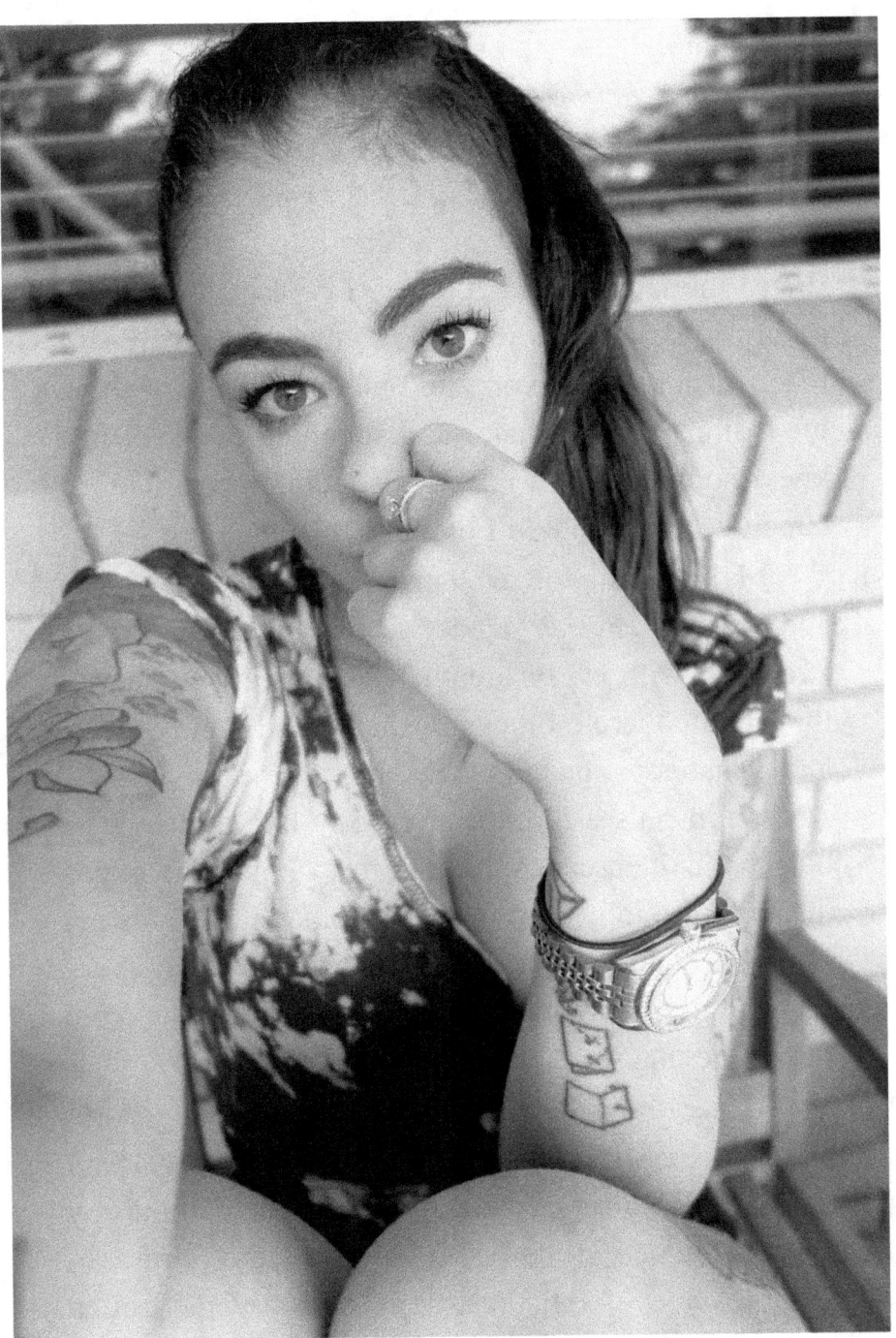

Dear Diary,

You ever wake up one day and think "What the fuck happened to me?" Of course, you do, you're me. I don't know what I expected being mentally ill would be like. But it was nothing like I imagined. At first, I thought there was a way I could make this all go away. I didn't know where to turn to for help so I reached out to everyone and anybody I could think of. I didn't know what was happening to me. I just knew something wasn't right. It didn't take long to conclude that I couldn't live like this anymore.

I know all too well the feeling of depression and overwhelming anxiety. It's like I'm being strangled with every breath I take. The weight of a thousand concrete blocks pushes down on my chest, and poisonous gas replaces the air in my lungs. Adrenalin pulses through my body like molten lava burning as it cascades through my veins. Fear surges through my body, knotting my stomach and twisting around my spine. Seeds of doubt get sown in every cell and grow into parasites that start eating me from the inside out.

Everything hurts. I feel like I am being burnt alive! I live in a state of constant dread. I am entombed in discomfort and apprehensive about my very existence. I suffer in silence, too afraid to speak. My eyes tell the truth, but everyone around has lost their sight. On the outside I am normal, but on the inside, I feel like an empty vessel. I am like a message in a bottle lost at sea. I bob up and down, aimlessly floating in the deep blue ocean. I can't stand to be inside myself, so I observe from afar. I am like a fly on the wall. When I look in the mirror, I can't help but wonder who that person is staring back at me. It doesn't look like me. A hideous, disgusting filthy creature no one should ever have to see. Who is this monster wearing my skin?

    I feel naked and vulnerable all the time. I can't go out in public because I can't stand the way they stare. Their eyes shoot red-hot hate and judgement like laser beams. In public, the feeling of being carefully watched is more intense, but it never seems to really end. The presence of extreme scrutiny is always in the air. Even when I am alone, the tiniest atoms in the atmosphere cut my skin like a million knives. Each breath I take feels like I am getting closer to death. The grim reaper's arrival always seems so imminent, but he never shows up. I can feel his presence, feel the scythe grazing my shoulder. I beg him to hook me, but he leaves, forcing me to endure another day.

    After a while, I become so exhausted it's like I'm floating. I am so weightless I wonder if I am still alive or whether I have died and gone to hell. It's like I'm living in a parallel dimension. Everyone moves around me, but I can't seem to interact with anyone.

I feel like I'm drowning. The end is near. I can feel the ringing in my ears. The waters are rising, the waves are crashing over me. Each one hits me like a knockout punch to the face. But I am so numb now I can't really feel a thing. I'm floating but sinking at the same time. It's like I'm always hovering just below the surface. I'm held down by an intense force that allows me to sip air as the water laps over my lips. I want to scream at the top of my lungs. But if I do, water will rush in.

I'm in so much pain I fear at any minute I'll die for real. I will be just another forgotten sailor lost in the seas of mental illness.

Sometimes the water is so murky even if I wanted to swim, I'm no longer sure which way is up. It's like I am always about to sink to the bottom, but I never seem to drown. The process of drowning goes on for so long, I am sure that at any minute it will kill me, but that's just it! It doesn't. It won't, it never will.

But I beg it to kill me, because what terrifies me more than the thought of drowning is the possibility that I will have to live like this for the rest of my life. Cursed to drift just below the waterline, never being able to rise or sink. Just floating, staring at the sun as it rises and falls each day wondering if I will ever be able to enjoy the new day it brings.

I spend my days drifting out at sea watching the birds fly above and the fish below, completely oblivious to me. It's as if I am underneath a glass coffee table where everyone else goes about their business, and I go unnoticed entombed in this glass coffin. People will tell me just to try to swim. But they don't see the invisible weight on my chest that's pinning me down. It's like I am paralysed and can't move my body. I can't swim either. I want to sink. I want the air to be emptied out of my lungs finally. I want to give my mind a chance to rest. But I can't. Everyone else seems to think that's a good thing. But I'm not so sure. They can't see what I see or feel the things I feel. They don't know what it's like to endure this hell day in, day out.

Nobody understands, and I don't expect them to. But I do expect them to believe me. Why are we all liars until proven otherwise? Isn't it innocent until proven guilty? Why does everyone automatically believe I am making it all up and not trying hard enough? Is my story more fanciful than the existence of God or aliens? Why do I have to prove my illness is real or that my symptoms exist? Mental illness is a thing, people! I thought we had established that already.

People want me to trust them with their advice and opinions, when they have no idea what they are talking about, but they judge and distrust my words when I speak from a heavy heart about what it's like to live inside my hell. I even had the typical, 'Think of all the people that have it so much worse than you' speech today. Excuse me for not giving a fuck about the people who have it worse than me today! In doing so I am not saying my struggle is worse than others. I am simply pointing out in my argument that they are trying to say my struggle is not significant. That type of thinking actually makes me suicidal.

If they were trying to cheer me up, then they failed miserably. They just made me feel worse, because now the ones I care about made it clear they don't give a fuck! They don't believe me, they don't understand, they don't care, and they don't even respect or value me enough to hear and listen to what I have to say. Worst of all, they then tell me how hard it is for them to see me struggle and make me feel like an asshole for even letting them see my struggle in the first place.

They say, "We are here for you." What they don't say is, "but we will make you feel like you are a burden on us and resent you for the rest of your days for making us a part of your life. But each time you need us, just ask so we can reassure you how much of an inconvenience you are on us."

I get made to feel like the boy who cried wolf all the time just for saying I'm not okay. After a while people just start to roll their eyes and say, "Yeah, we know. You already said that. We are sick of hearing about it. Say something more positive next time." Then I just feel bad for inconveniencing them. So now I just stay quiet. No one wants to hear it. So why should I waste my breath speaking it?

Silenced Barbie

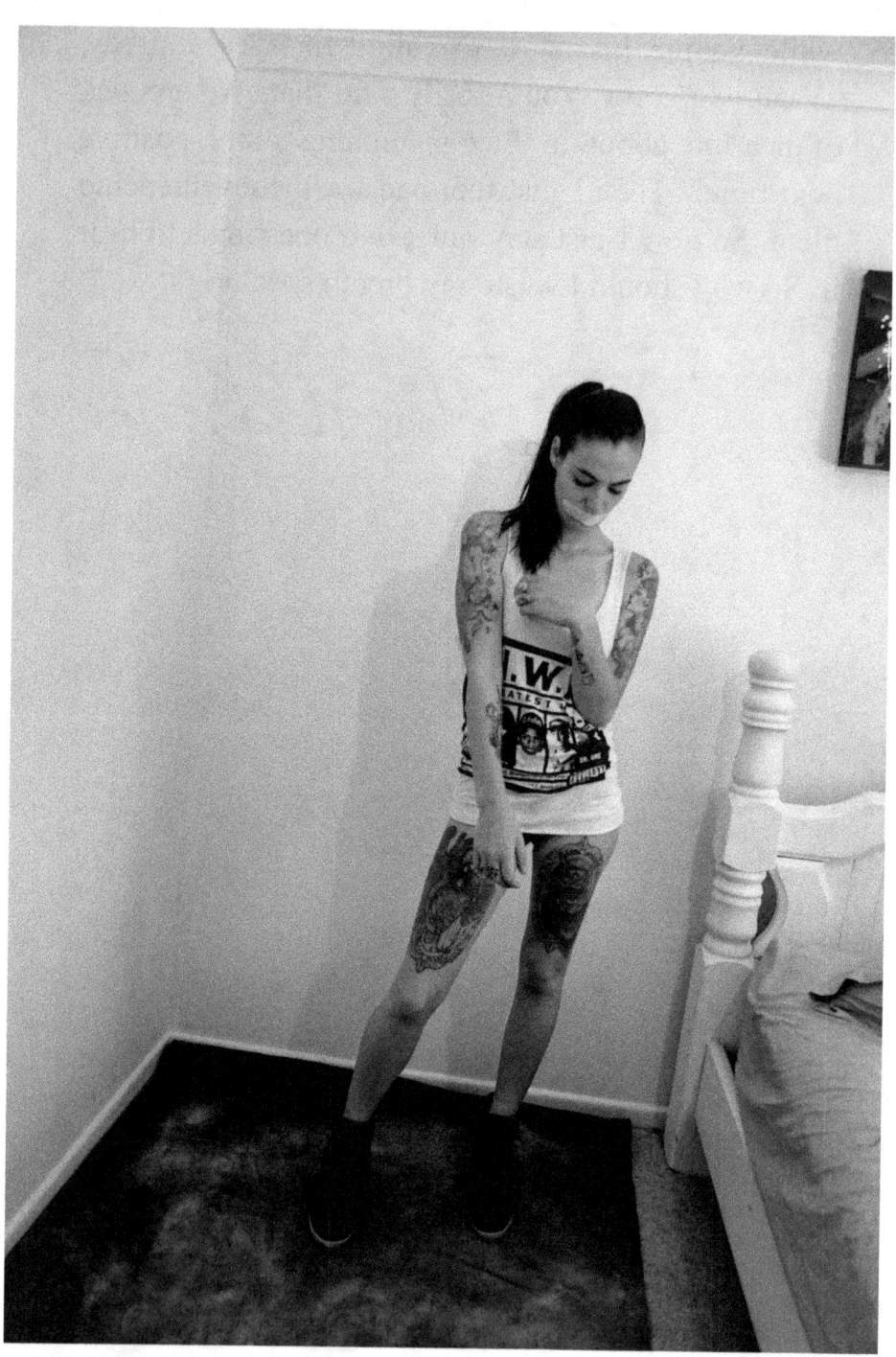

Dear Diary,

There's a hell of a lot I have to be upset about right now. I feel a lot of resentment, a considerable amount of doubt and frustration towards others, myself and my situation. The list of the things I have every right to complain about is endless. The injustices I suffer at the hands of the legal, government and medical systems are just the beginning. Society's social norms seem to give others a right to discriminate against me.

I have a crippling illness that makes keeping myself alive an almost impossible feat. An illness that makes the most basic things like sleeping and eating extremely difficult at times. Symptoms like fatigue, nausea, migraines and insomnia interfere with every aspect of my life. It severely interferes with my quality of life, making living pure hell at times. But I don't think about that. There's no point. I can't change any of it.

So what do I focus on? I focus on what I can change, the challenges at hand and the choices I have, on making the most of the bad situation I am in. Lying in bed for days is no good when I don't have a house to live in. My favourite coping mechanism, avoidance, is no good when I have to support myself financially. If I can't leave my house, then I can't get to work. If I don't get to work, I have no money, which means my bills don't get paid and very soon I won't even have a house to avoid going to work in. There's no one to pick up the pieces and clean up my mess if I don't.

So I get out my broom and sweep it all up. I pull myself together because falling apart is a luxury I cannot afford. I function, but barely. I function because I have to. I do it so well that people assume I'm doing okay when I'm really not.

I feel the tears well in my eyes as I pick up my shield – like Captain America – and prepare for another fight. I try to eliminate distractions so that I can focus on survival; it's all I seem to do these days. Survival is my baseline. Life is hard. Life is unfair. People judge me for my downward spirals. But I am trying so hard to keep my head above water. It's a slippery slope that I keep tripping into. It's like trying to hold onto a bar of soap in a prison toilet. The harder you cling to it, the more slippery it gets. Eventually you are going to get fucked.

I cling to my sanity like a dog latching onto a bone. I am hanging from a single strand of rope above a large ravine. I am a thousand meters off the ground watching the rope fray more and more each time I sway. They fail to see what I see that I could be falling faster. I could at any moment fall apart, break and disappear like a magician right before their eyes. All they see are the thousands of escape acts Houdini successfully performed. But I live in fear of the one time I can't pull off the unbelievable trick. I defy the odds every day just to live.

It's extremely hard to find the strength to persevere when you are only going backwards in life. But what else can I do?

Avoidance Barbie

Falling into water doesn't kill you. It's not being able to get out that makes you drown.

Bipolar Barbie

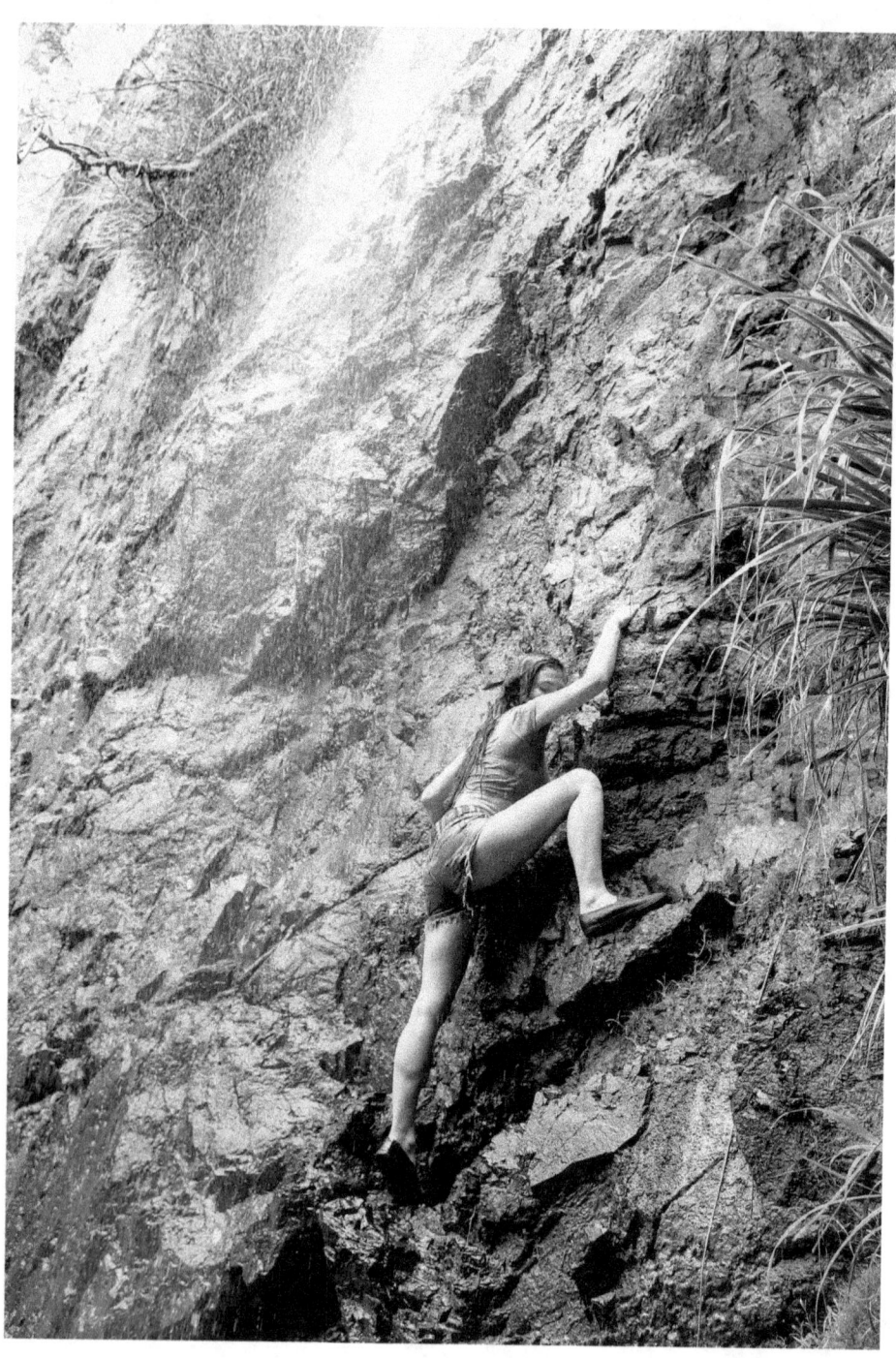

Dear Diary,

    I am tormented day and night by the demons that hide inside my mind. I am trapped inside a world I can't seem to get out of. Voices calling out, "cut me" as I stare at my arm. "Let it bleed," they whisper as I hold my head up high and try to ignore the thoughts tugging at me.

    I am alive, I know that. But sometimes I wish I were dead. There's this unbearable feeling I just can't seem to shake. It's like I am being burnt alive. I am a witch being persecuted at the stake. I feel like someone is holding a welding torch to my skin. I can't bear this torture. Each day I live I am in more pain.

    There's a wave perched above my head. I live in fear every second of every day, with it looming above me. I am anxiously awaiting the moment it finally happens. The moment it all comes crashing down, and I drown. Drowning would be a blessing. "Put me out of this misery," I beg; I can't stand the thought of another day like today.

    Each glance from a stranger in the street cuts me like razor blades. I feel their judgement burning holes into my skin. I squirm, there's no escape. I feel like I'm stuck in a cage as I pull the doona covers over my head. I lay here in fear, curled up as tight as I can. I feel if I glance around the corner, behind my bedroom door, I'll see the beast that lays in wait ready to devour me whole.

I have nothing left to fight this beast off but my bare hands. I shiver in pure terror. I fear for my life. Who am I kidding, this is just another day in my life. A nightmare I can't seem to wake from. It's *Groundhog Day*. I am stuck in a time loop, year after year, the same patterns, the same routines. I am cursed. Can it be reversed? Is there an antidote for this poison I must have consumed? When will it take my life?

I just want to die. I've been sitting too long in the desert on this pinnacle as high as the clouds in the sky. It's so thin and steep I sit up here like a bird on a perch too scared to move. I am terrified of heights. I try not to look down. This ledge is just round enough to sit up on it, but I can still touch the sides all the way around. I feel the rocks fall away as my fingers fiddle for a better grip. The tiny stones crumbling from this ledge ricochet off the sides of this vast cavern like bullets raining down on a mobster's house. I listen carefully, but it's so high I never hear them hit the ground. The hole goes straight down.

I've sat up here so long I've come to the only logical conclusion, my only way down is to jump. Certain death awaits, but uncertain death is coming too. As my flesh is picked raw by the vultures. I am exposed and vulnerable. I am used and abused as they swoop down on me and pick me apart. Sensing my weakened state they devour whatever is left of my tattered carcass.

I scream, but no one hears me. I lost hope of a rescue many years ago. It seems that I am perceived as nothing more than a spectacle. Others watch in awe, offering guilt and shame. I am hanging centre stage, right in the middle of the Grand Canyon and busloads of people come to take my picture. But no one knows the true extent of the danger I am in. Most assume it is a carefully planned stunt.

Some days I feel so alone in the bitter cold. But when the sun is scorching hot, it seems I am a magnet for a very unreceptive crowd. It is not my intention to put on a show. Their feedback is given freely, but their help comes at a price.

I wonder if they would forgive me if I jumped? Or would they tell me I should have suffered longer?

Wounded Barbie

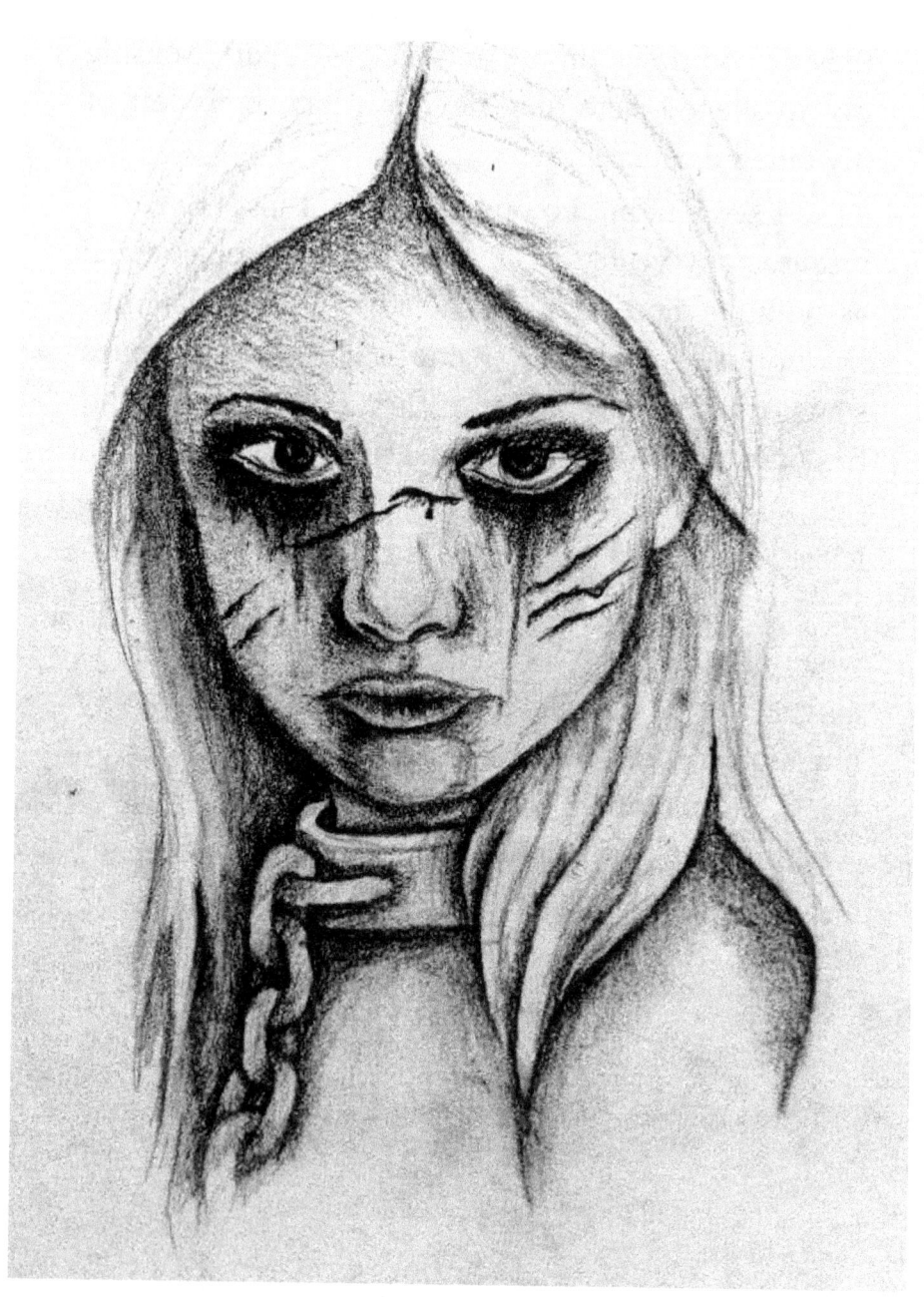

Dear Diary,

Today can be summed up in three words. "I can't breathe"

It might not seem like I am about to asphyxiate but you don't need water to drown or lack of air to suffocate. Self-doubt can do it for you without a single sound. Just the quickened rhythm of my heart overbeating, and my shallow breath. The tightness in my chest is compressed more with each weak, whistled breath. Every terrible moment of my life is compacted, filling me with a density I can no longer withstand.

It seems that no matter how quickly I learn to swim, it never seems fast enough. The darkness is like quicksand. It latches onto me, and won't let go. I am trying to just go about my life like none of this ever happened. I try to just live my life like everyone else wants me to. But it's too hard. I am losing my mind with concern for my own wellbeing. But then again do I really care what happens to me? I must, because why else would I still be here? I am reckless though. I do push the envelope a little too far when it comes to living life on the edge. I guess that's what happens when you are teetering on the edge of reality. Why restrict yourself to the rules of life and death when you are not even sure you are still living?

Why has my relationship with mortality

changed so drastically? Sometimes I welcome my own demise, but when I don't, I just accept it as a murderous shadow that could attack at any moment. I know it's there. I am even friendly towards it. Sometimes I invite him in for a glass of wine and some sleeping pills, painkillers or *Valium*. Other times I just let him watch me when I sleep. Sometimes he embraces me like a partner giving me comfort in my time of need. He promises safety, a solution and an end to my suffering. He is at times my best friend and other times my annoying neighbour.

There's a muddle of emotions that have come together to create one big lump that sits in the back of my throat. They melt in the cauldron of my stomach where confusion, anger, guilt, doubt, melancholy and self-hatred all mix together forming a formidable potion. The effect is a state I call my darkest depression. I'm so low I can't see anything but the darkness of a pitch black moonless night. It's like I've fallen off the edge of a cliff into the ocean at night with no flashlight. I'm stuck in the whitewash as the waves crash down on me, pinning me under and slamming me against the sharp, jagged rocky edge. I can't breathe. I tumble and tumble as I am thrashed about, against my will. I am becoming increasingly more terrified. I am afraid that I will never get out!

I relate to the whitewash beating against the rocks as I watch my boyfriend fish. He isn't much of a talker on these fishing trips, despite dragging me along. I guess this is his interpretation of "quality time". Since our relationship began I have spent hundreds of hours watching the ferocious ocean smash against the shore. Rain, hail or shine, he drags me out here when I can't find another excuse. When I do, he uses guilt trips to get me to cancel my plans and accompany him anyway.

I watch the ocean become deceptively calm before surging again. The water is sucked back into its mass before gathering in a large mountain of water to pound the jagged rocks. During the lulls, I watch a fisherman cast his line, patiently awaiting a nibble or a bite. He waits for the sinker to hit the bottom as his reel whirs away. He waits in anticipation for the moment he gets to flick the reel and lock the bail, adjusting the drag until he seems satisfied he has found the ideal position to catch a fish. Or so I guess his logic goes. I follow his actions and movements with my eyes but my mind creates a different narrative. I find myself wishing I was a heavy lead sinker on the end of a fishing line, so that I could sink to the bottom and drown.

As he turns to look back at me perched on the highest rock, I wonder if he knows I am thinking about dying when we exchange pleasant smiles? I muster a smile back and try not to look suicidal or insanely bored. I don't even know if I would call it boredom. There is just something about this suffocating heaviness that makes doing things irrelevant. I am not even sure I am still existing anymore. Sometimes I have to pinch myself just to check that I am still alive. I feel like I am petrified, perched up here on this rock like a gargoyle. I squat on the edge of the ledge rocking back and forth hugging my legs close to my chest and resting my weary head on my knees. I guess I space out a lot.

Sometimes I travel in my mind to the life I think I should be living. Sometimes I travel to the past. Sometimes I fast forward to the future where I can imagine a brighter version of me and my life. Sometimes I just relive the worst moments of my life over and over again until I am properly traumatised. Sometimes I even create *new* worst moments. I play out the deaths of everyone I care about, I watch them die, I attend their funerals, I grieve for them and all the while I smile, nod my head and act like I am listening to someone else recount how some jerk cut them off in traffic. #SanePeopleProblems

I am not sure whether or not I would call it a compulsion or an obsession. The scenarios are fabricated by some deep dark version of me. I am in control of my fate in my own imagination. The genre depends on my mood on that particular day. It could be a light-hearted romantic comedy, inspirational story, superhero movie or *The Conjuring*. Most days it's a mixture of recurring themes from every piece of traumatising entertainment I have ever seen or heard about. Does that make me a sadist? Is it true that I want to wallow in my own self-pity? Do I secretly want to be like this? Do I get some sick satisfaction out of it?

Personally I think my mind is just trying to come to terms with my emotions. My wild imagination is trying to justify the existence of my feelings, i.e. the only reason someone should feel this terrible is if something terrible had *actually* happened. It rationalises these intense, irrational and disproportionate feelings of gore by creating its own justification.

If my own brain can't believe it, then perhaps there really is no hope of proving it to others?

Suicidal Barbie

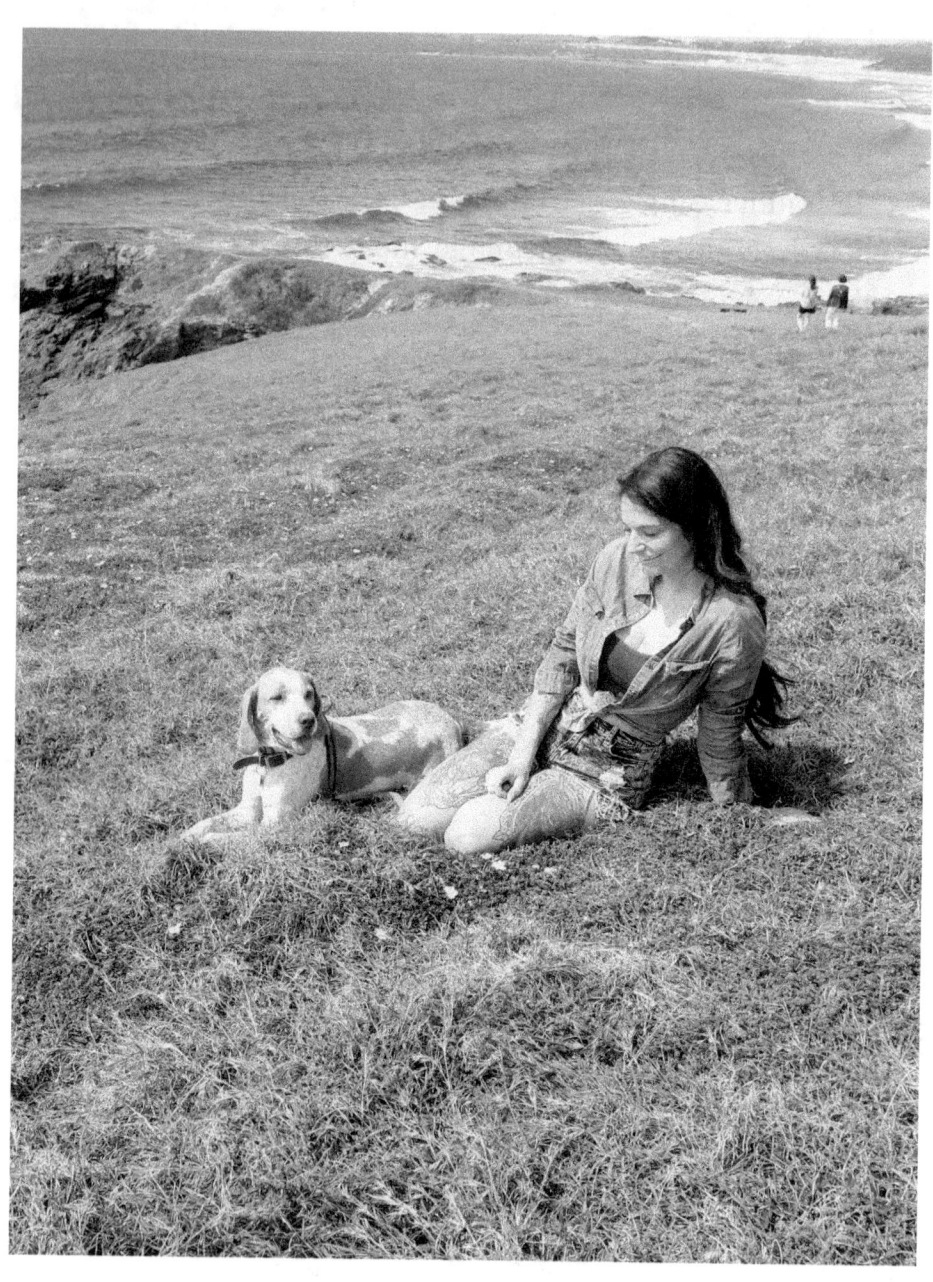

Dear Diary,

My housemate commented on the state of my room, and I realise it is in a pretty disgusting state at the moment. It is both messy and dirty. I have found it difficult to just keep up with everyday things. I am all over the place. I am not bad. In fact, I am good. I'm great! But that's just it. I know Bipolar Disorder is not as simple as Depression. With Depression, recovery is happiness. That is not an accurate gauge of Bipolar Disorder recovery because to me, happiness is manic euphoria.

I know the dangers of being "happy". But I am fine. I really am. I am just such a perfectionist in myself and know too much about my illness that I am constantly assessing where I am at. The trouble is, where I am at changes so quickly, days, hours, weeks, months. I am constantly switching but also constantly evolving. My doctors tell me they have never seen the same person twice in our consults. Not always because of my illness. But because my brain works with such speed, I am constantly evolving as I understand the world around me. I process difficult concepts in minutes. Each new encounter, each new experience I absorb everything I can to learn from it. My brain is thirsty for knowledge and answers.

I have been investigating the world around me and within me since the day I was born. 'A child with a curious mind', they labelled me. I was always watching, observing and pondering. I have spent hours, days and weeks on my best friend's couch and she observes me sometimes. She knows me too well. She can see my mind ticking over. Careful not to disturb, she waits, assuming I will turn to her and reveal my deepest thoughts. But sometimes I don't. She knows my mind is vast, cavernous, perhaps even endless.

A lot of people think they know me because I share a lot of myself with basically everyone. But I feel the need to remind people who read my blogs that if you think you know everything about me, you are wrong. I have come to learn that the more you think you know about someone, the less you actually do. Those who read my blogs only know the tip of the iceberg. There's not enough time in this life to divulge every thought, action or contemplation I may have. I have far too many. My mind never stops. The cogs are constantly turning like a clock wound up way too far. I absorb too much information from the world around me to be able to process it myself, let alone explain it to someone else.

I feel like I am always trying to explain to people why I hit the iceberg as if I was the captain of the Titanic. All I know for sure is that a captain must go down with his ship and I am sinking rapidly. The water is rushing in and I don't have a bucket large enough to bail the water out. I am no longer the captain. I am Jack, handcuffed to a pole below deck. The water is up to my neck! "I am sinking!" I scream, but everyone else has already abandoned the ship.

I am alone; sinking to the bottom of the ocean, facing my intimate doom. I feel like I am hyper aware of everything inside myself. I have been told time and time again my self-awareness has been my salvation. I think it is also my undoing. I need time in solitude to process it all.

In the beginning I was being pulled to the bottom so fast that I could not comprehend what had happened. It was as if someone had filled my pockets with stones that weighed me down and held me under. I quickly learnt that kicking, straining and flailing my arms about in a desperate manner was only going to tire me out. No matter how hard I tried to go up, the only direction I seemed to travel was further downward. Terror began to set in when I realized that I was only descending deeper into the bottomless ocean of depression.

I searched with anguish for a single reason to continue this tiresome battle. It was as if depression was a sea monster that I had to defeat before I could be deemed worthy to return to the surface. I was Ariel, the little mermaid desperately wanting to return to land. But whatever was holding me down was a relentless force unwilling to release its grasp. The longer I stayed in the darkness, the less light I could see coming from the surface. As the light inside me faded, so did my ambition to survive.

People think analysing yourself is a choice. I call it human nature. Anyone who doesn't analyse themselves is going against our primal programming. Perhaps I am alone in that belief. "Just stop thinking," they advise. I try, but I can never seem to turn my brain off. I think a lot, but I wouldn't call it 'overthinking'. The classic definition of 'overthinking' is to think about something too much or for too long. I am of the opinion that I think just the right amount. If you ask me, I believe the rest of the world thinks much too little. It's only a problem when you can't get out of your own head. I wouldn't say that I can't, more that I just don't want to.

It's not all worrying. A lot of it is scientific discovery. That's who I am. That's what I do. I have never done things any differently. I observe, analyse, wonder, theorise and explore the most probable possibilities by comparing them all in a millisecond. Things make logical sense to me in a way many others just can't seem to understand.

When I got sick – or at least the moment I realised something was seriously wrong with me – that's how I automatically dealt with it. I tried to solve the problem. The trouble was, I didn't know exactly what the dilemma was. I thought I found the answers, but then I just found a million more questions.

I hate talking about my illness, my diagnosis, sickness, disease, mental illness and mental health or whatever the fuck you want to call it. I just wish we had a few more words. I mean it's all very ambiguous. I think it over generalises the subject and just gets old really fast. Not to mention some people get on their high horse and start galloping at me wanting to joust over the use of those words. What else am I meant to call it? I can't think of any other way to refer to it. Maybe that's the only problem I can't solve, and it's driving me mad!

I can do anything when I put my mind to it. Anything except magically cure myself. I wish I had Cinderella's fairy godmother or a magic mirror on the wall. Fuck the ball, I just want to be normal after all.

What more can a girl wish for?

Overthinking Barbie

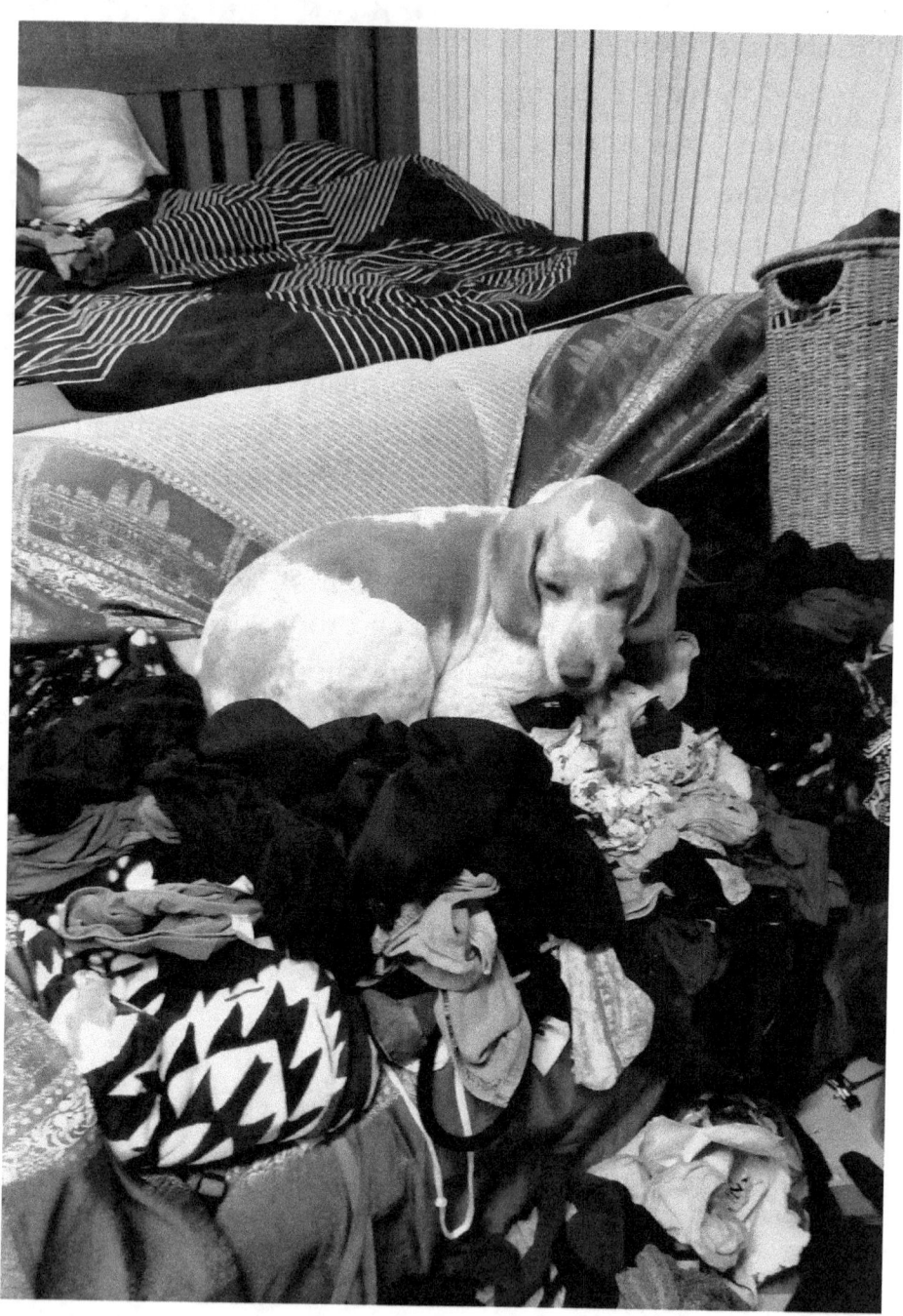

Dear Diary,

I broke down last night. I didn't even see it coming. I was outside having a cigarette, and I just fell to the floor. I couldn't stand up. I started crying, and I couldn't stop. I curled up in a ball on the floor, and all I could think was, "I can't do this anymore! I can't do this, I can't do this, I can't do this, I can't do this." The thoughts played on repeat in a tormented loop.

It's not from lack of trying. I work so hard every day. But is there a point where someone becomes so broken they can't be glued back together? What happens to Humpty Dumpty when all the king's horses and all the king's men leave? I don't even know where to begin putting all the pieces back together. I wonder how long they tried. Did they just grow tired after a while? If they had tried every day for the rest of their lives would poor Humpty still be alive?

It seems like it's a race against the clock. It's just a matter of time before I'm a cracked egg cooking on the searing pavement. It seems like I'm falling apart faster than I can put myself back together. I'm falling as I have been for years, but I don't seem to be getting anywhere this time. It seems like my insides have been pulled apart too many times to count. It's like each time I have to do it, there are less pieces to pick up this time round. Each time I break I leave a piece of me behind.

I would give anything to feel like the girl that went to her first day of school full of excitement and energy. But now, it's all gone, all drained out of me like a tap with no water left in the pipes.

Who will catch me if I fall, alone, in my backyard at night? I assume the answer is no one. No one will catch me if I fall because no one sees me falling. I don't speak about it; I don't talk about it because no one wants to hear it. They have made that very clear. There's still the ignorant idiots that try to convince me I'm not falling. They think that makes me wrong, but in truth, it shows how blind they really are to the truth. Everyone seems to want to help me find the light. But what if there is no light?

What if I died tonight?

Suicidal Barbie

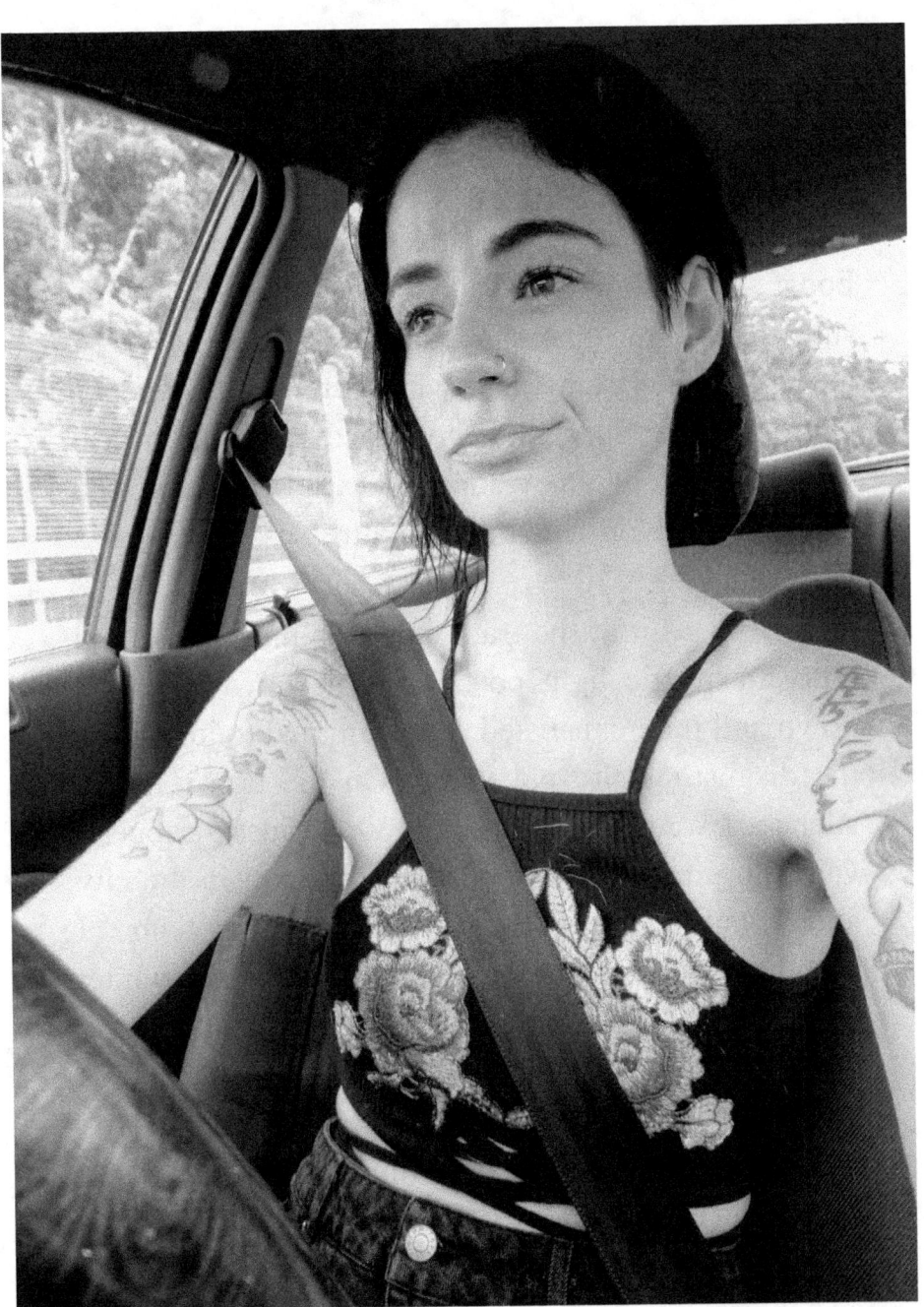

Dear Diary,

Today I forced myself to function. Well, I guess that depends on what you call 'functioning'. I got up, and I went to work. The extra medication I am taking for my depression has given me a slight boost. Just enough to walk I guess. But everything rubs against me like sandpaper. My head is heavy, and I feel like I am filled with water. I just want to sink into the floor like the Wicked Witch in *The Wizard of Oz*. I am restless like the princess who tried to sleep on a hundred mattresses on top of a pea.

As I wait at the tram stop this morning I hold onto the traffic light post. There is nowhere to sit down and I am exhausted. I am tempted to just sit on the disgusting city pavement. On the tram I sit in silence. I want to be invisible. Or to just disappear, vanishing into thin air. I get off the tram in the city and I walk through the crowded shopping centre. I withdraw beneath the large hood of my red winter coat. I try to blend in and hold my head low. My mother tells me I slouch. Well, I'm trying to be as small as I can be. I don't want to be here; I don't want to be anywhere.. Bed sounds like the place to be. I don't want anyone to see me today. I can't muster a smile on my face or the energy to greet customers. I hope no one talks to me at work today, I don't have the energy to function. It would be best if

I wasn't here. Each second I am, the anxiety grows and my heart begins to race.

I have tunnel vision. There's a black cloud around my head. I feel my body cave in on itself. I am here, but nobody is home. I am somewhere else. Where? I do not know. I am not present in this realm as depression takes hold. Life just seems to get in the way. Why can't I just shrink away and disappear? I am cold in the air conditioning, shivering in fact. I am wearing a jumper, but I think the cold is echoing from my soul. I am somewhere in hell, sometimes it burns like volcanic fire and other times I am frozen in the dead of night. I am feverish with sadness and grief. The shivers come and go.

I have lost all the energy to pretend that I am okay, because the truth is that I'm not; it's about time somebody knew. The trouble with letting people know is that they assume it only began at the time I told them when in truth, I've been struggling for years. The past couple of months have been some of the worst months yet. There hasn't been a minute in this past week where I haven't been moments away from calling an ambulance and checking myself into the public inpatient ward. But I don't because honestly, I am terrified. I have heard nothing but horrible stories of that place and they are so strict; there's no smoking, no coffee, no phones, no computers, no TV, no leaving, absolutely nothing. I think if I was locked up in a hospital without those things – including my dog, Northy – I would become insane (if I'm not already).

I spend countless hours in bed wondering what it would be like to be hospitalised. I have private health insurance, but I am waiting for the waiting period to end so I can be admitted to the private psych ward. What will I do without Northy though? What will I do without my partner? How will I survive there? I am scared. I don't want to be tied to a bed or forced to take meds. But then again, I do want to be better and I would do anything for that.

I'll decide I'm going to do it one minute, because the day gets so bad I begin to scream for help. Then the next minute, the fear kicks in, and I'll decide not to do it. I am constantly swinging back and forth convincing myself I need help and then convincing myself I can do it on my own. So instead I spend days at home wondering how my life has reached this point. How did I end up like this? Why did the darkness decide to settle in me?

How can I get rid of it?

Depressed Barbie

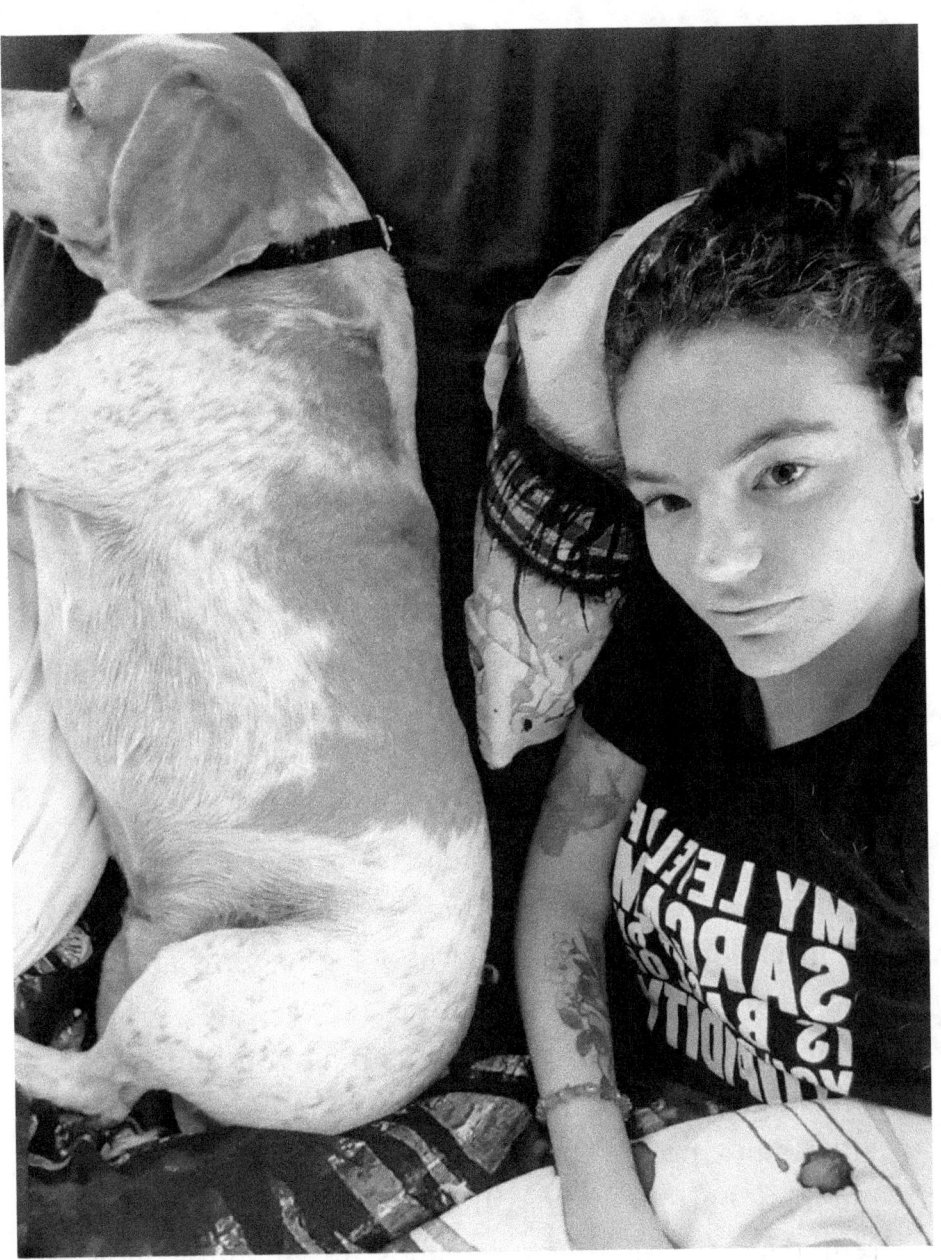

Dear Diary,

I feel like a liar when I tell people I'm busy. I always seem to be working but have no idea what I do with my time. In truth I was busy. But not in the way most people would define the word. As far as the dictionary definition goes, having a great deal to do and keeping oneself occupied is being busy. I certainly have a lot to do, taming my wild thoughts. That certainly keeps me occupied for extended periods, if not every waking hour of my day.

What people don't understand is how involved being mentally ill is. If you are actively trying to recover then you will have twenty-four hours a day, seven days a week concerned for your mental wellbeing. That part comes pretty naturally to me. But it's what you do with that time that really counts.

I try to learn as much as I can so that I'm fighting subconsciously even when my conscious brain is not. I use my mind like a sponge to absorb every bit of information. You never know when something might be critical in helping you figure out what's going on. I don't always remember all of it, but I am a pretty absorbent sponge. You can wring me out, but there is still a lot of dampness that remains. Mental illness demands my attention most hours of the day, and when I don't give in it takes over! People accuse me of being consumed by my thoughts, and while that may be true, I did not let that happen willingly. I can sit at home and do nothing and be busy all day. I could lay in bed all day and still be run off my feet.

Even when I am functioning, I am working overtime. I am always trying to be in two places at once, in my mind and everywhere else outside. It follows me around like a bad smell. I can't just shake it off. It's one of those dense farts that lingers in your personal space you can't just subtly waft away. It's thick and takes forever to disperse. There are too many particles to be diluted effectively by the air around you.

Distraction can help, but sometimes you have no hope. People expect you to do things. They are always saying, "Come on, do this. Now! You're doing nothing ..."

FUCK OFF! I am doing *everything*! You just can't see it! I'm in bed because I am fighting a war in my head! I am exhausted. I need a break but lying in bed isn't a break. Sorry, I couldn't come to your barbeque, I have no excuse other than I needed some time to myself. I didn't want it, but I couldn't do more than the enormous amount of work I was doing in my head. Just because I went to work today doesn't mean I'm fine! It was excruciatingly painful to have to function at work and silence my mind all day. Now that I get home I am under siege by my angry mind fighting for control. Now my thoughts are super pissed off that I've ignored them all day. They start yelling at me, demanding my attention. "Get out!" I scream at the thoughts, but they refuse to leave.

    I wish people would stop calling me lazy. They have no idea what I'm dealing with! Despite how horrific mental illness makes me feel, what hurts the most is knowing that everyone thinks I am making it all up. Depressed people are apparently all lazy liars that just don't want to work hard. Do people actually think we enjoy being this way? The stigma really gets under my skin. I can see how it would appear that way to others who are incredibly ignorant, but the truth is, by the time I have gotten through all the shit in my head each morning, I am already in a bad mood. I am too exhausted to function before I ever really began my day

    Mental illness is not an excuse. But it might be a very valuable explanation when I'm angry and frustrated with myself because I just can't do all the things I want to do. I think not only do we have to acknowledge that mental illness is real, but that the struggles and setbacks we face are real too. So that people are not just accepting of the idea of mental health, but that they are also understanding of and tolerant towards the impact that it may have on someone's life. Then maybe we won't be so judgemental about where we are at in life or what we can and can't do. Perhaps we will start to be proud of the effort people living with mental illness actually put into keeping themselves alive.

If my mind was a business and my thoughts were people, everyone would be saying to me, "just close the doors! You can't work every second of every day twenty-four hours a day, seven days a week! You need a holiday! You need to hire more staff! Lessen your workload!" But my mentally ill mind doesn't have a closing time, I don't have any staff to help me, and I can't escape the 24/7 onslaught. Yes I know with therapy and meds and blah blah bullshit it all helps, and I do that! But I want to bring awareness to what we have to overcome first, because people can't see this invisible illness; they don't acknowledge its existence. "Get a job you bum!" They cry. "Get off your ass and do something for once! Stop being so lazy all the time! You do nothing! Why are you so exhausted and tired all the time!" I feel guilty every time I cancel plans for no better reason than I can't get a hold of my mind.

The reality of it is ... I do a hell of a lot before I even start my real life. I have come to learn that real life is a luxury. It's non-existent until you deal with your mind. That's why I take my meds, go to therapy and work 24/7 to research, educate myself and explore ways to deal with my mind. So that one day I might only be living one life. *My* life. Mental illness free!

Only once I stop living to survive can I actually start *living*. My focus can then be about more than just getting through each day. I can one day live a fulfilling life. Isn't that what we all dream about?

Lazy Barbie

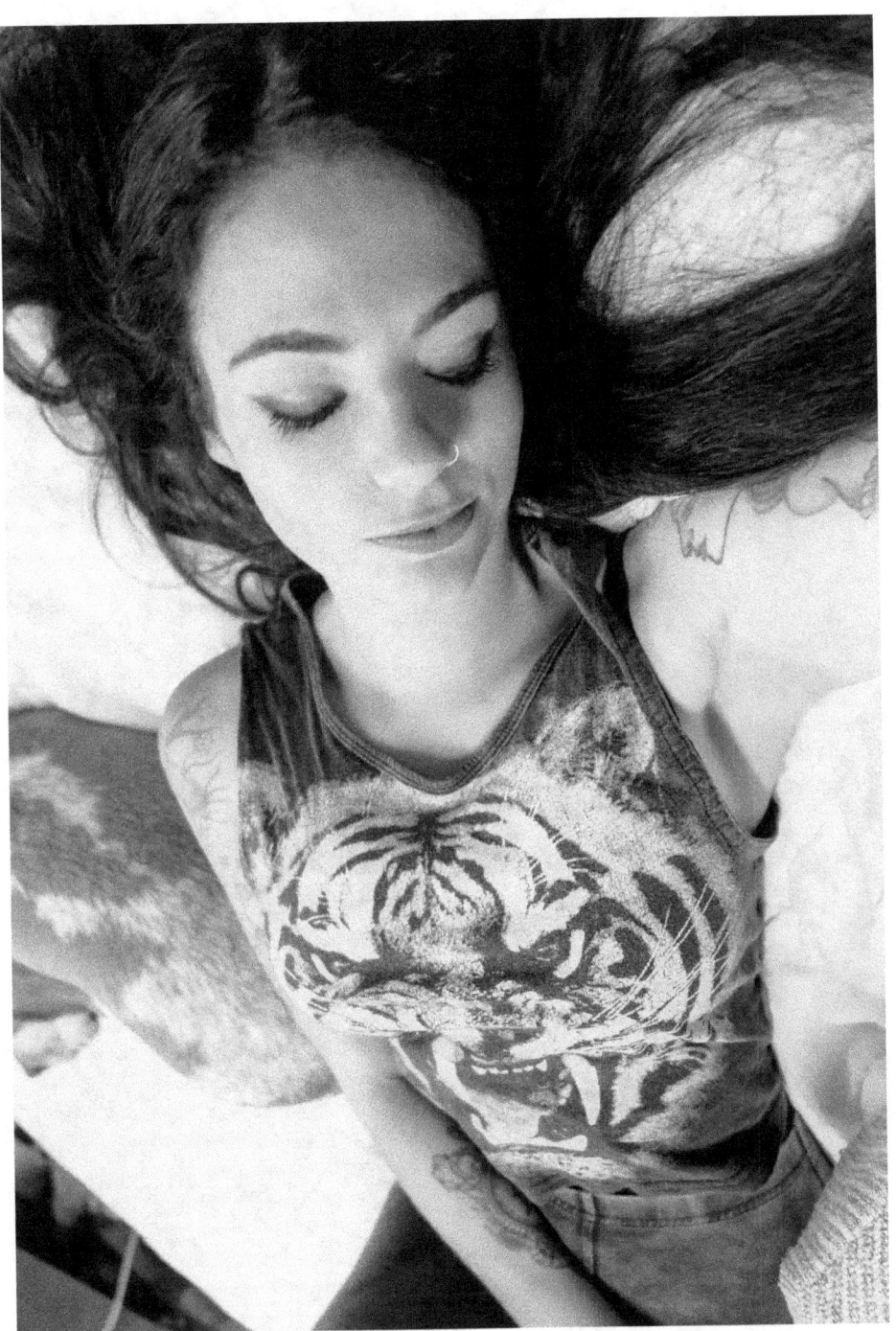

The saddest things is that people truly believed that I deliberately drowned

Bipolar Barbie

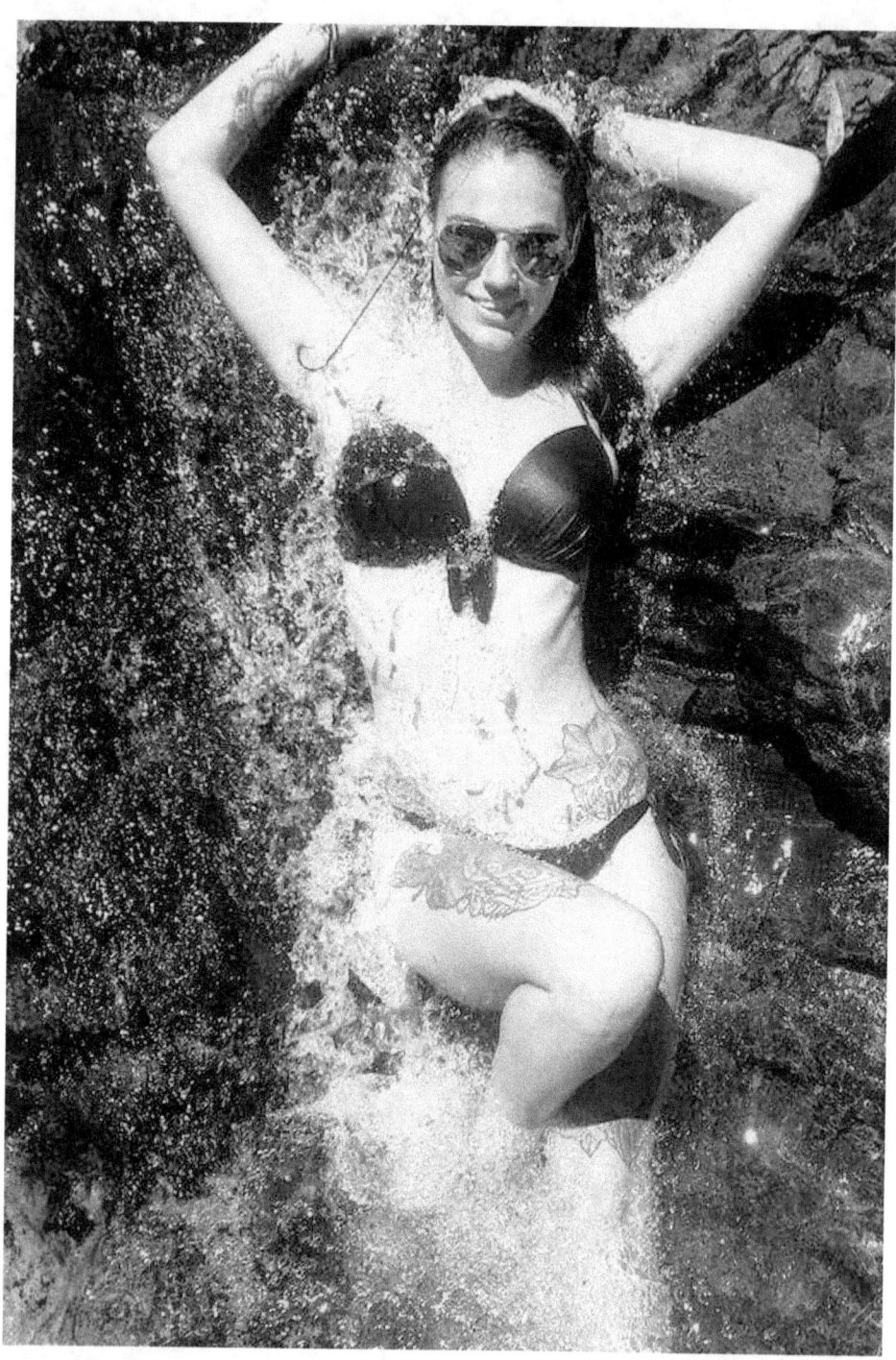

Dear Diary,

The only thing that compares to the pain of losing yourself is the fact that people feel the need to tell you it was all your fault. It's like if they don't, then they think it's automatically their fault or something. It's no one's fault really.

I guess no one wants to believe something so horrific can happen with no rhyme or reason. It's a terrifying concept that anyone could lose their mind at any moment without warning. I understand that … it's even more frightening to realise it's happening to you.

I wish people could see past their reduced opinions of my struggle to at least acknowledge that. I get it must be hard for them to witness, but do they really think it was less difficult to live? I watched my life fall apart, and my world go up in flames too! I watched it burn around me like in a blazing inferno that even Dante would not believe existed.

I have picked myself up time and time again hoping it would be the last time. But I've always been a clumsy person. The trouble is … I have no idea what I am tripping over. My own feet? I have spent so many years in the darkness without anything to light my way. "Just leave that place," they all said. What the fuck do they think I have been trying to do?

Everyone is quick to point out how I seem to have lost my way. But I haven't just lost my way. For a long time, there was no way out. I was caged like an animal. I desperately tried to free myself, to run from myself, but that was never going to work. I was like Little Red Riding Hood running through the woods, hiding from the Big Bad Wolf we call depression. I have been leaving bread crumbs like Hansel and Gretel for others to find me. But I am about to be boiled alive and no one has found me. I am scared. The worst part is … I no longer know who the witch is. Is it me? Could they be right? Am I the villain in this story? Am I the reason why I suffer so much? Is this a curse or a spell I am casting on myself? Why does everyone treat me like the boy who cried wolf? Why do I have to prove I am in danger to receive help?

They might not see it, but I am standing on the edge of a cliff, about to jump or even just fall to my death. Both are a possibility. It's not just a metaphor. The other night I walked all the way to the quarry. I sat as close to the edge as my fear of heights allowed me and I drank a bottle of tequila. I wanted to know what it would feel like if I jumped. I wanted to know if I would change my mind. My fear of heights did save me on that night. But there are many other ways I can take my life.

It blows my mind how I can be at uni all day

and no one knows what I get up to when no one is watching. I observe my friends in the dining room laughing and sharing innocent stories. I sit in silence, half listening to their conversations. Half wondering how they will react to the news I am dead. Will they mourn my loss for long? Or at all? How will I be remembered? Sometimes they interrupt my absent poise. But most of the time they just carry on like I am not even there. I watch them carefully and feel no emotion at all. I am numb. I try to smile; I try to laugh. Sometimes I even do.

I wonder if they know it's all an act. My parents think my sadness is an act. *This* is what feels like an act: getting up and going to class when I am on my deathbed. This act is the greatest challenge I have ever faced. I feel like I am in a never-ending Shakespearean play. The script is longer than Homer's Odyssey. I hope this feeling doesn't last as long as the siege of Troy. I don't have time for that. It isn't part of my five-year plan.

The whole reason I applied to study at this university was because of their accelerated programs. I already feel like I am behind, graduating high school at nineteen years old. I took that gap year to Germany when I was sixteen, and while I do not regret that choice, I am now twenty and failing classes. All of my classmates are two or three years younger than me. I feel like time is something I don't have. Time passes so slow as each second drags on. It seems to be slipping through my fingers as each day and week blurs into the next.

I feel like I am starring in my own movie. There's a camera behind me and it just follows me around. I feel like the world is a screen. Everything is two dimensional. I am scared I have detached myself from reality. Everything around me feels like a movie set. Everyone seems to be playing a role . Can they really be that happy? Why do they seem to actually enjoy being alive? I don't get it. I'm running from life. I am afraid of reality. What is life if you can't stand to live it? Why is everything so hard?

I am running away from life and everything it entails. I just want to escape this suffocating feeling that is gripping me tightly in its unrelenting grasp. I feel like the Big Bad Wolf is chasing me through the woods.

I can't help but wonder, is this what life is meant to be? Hard and sad? It felt like it was before, but now I know that it can't be true. Life can't mean this much pain, right? No one deserves to suffer every day! Every hour feels worse than the last and there's no end in sight. The only way out of the pain is death and I'm tired of trying to fight against something so strong when all hope seems to be lost.

Feelings of dread, regret and sorrow flood my body and overload it like a computer. My brain freezes and my entire system seems to be failing. I am paralysed by fear. The only thoughts I can seem to maintain is the acceptance of my death. No one is coming to save me.

Red Riding Hood Barbie

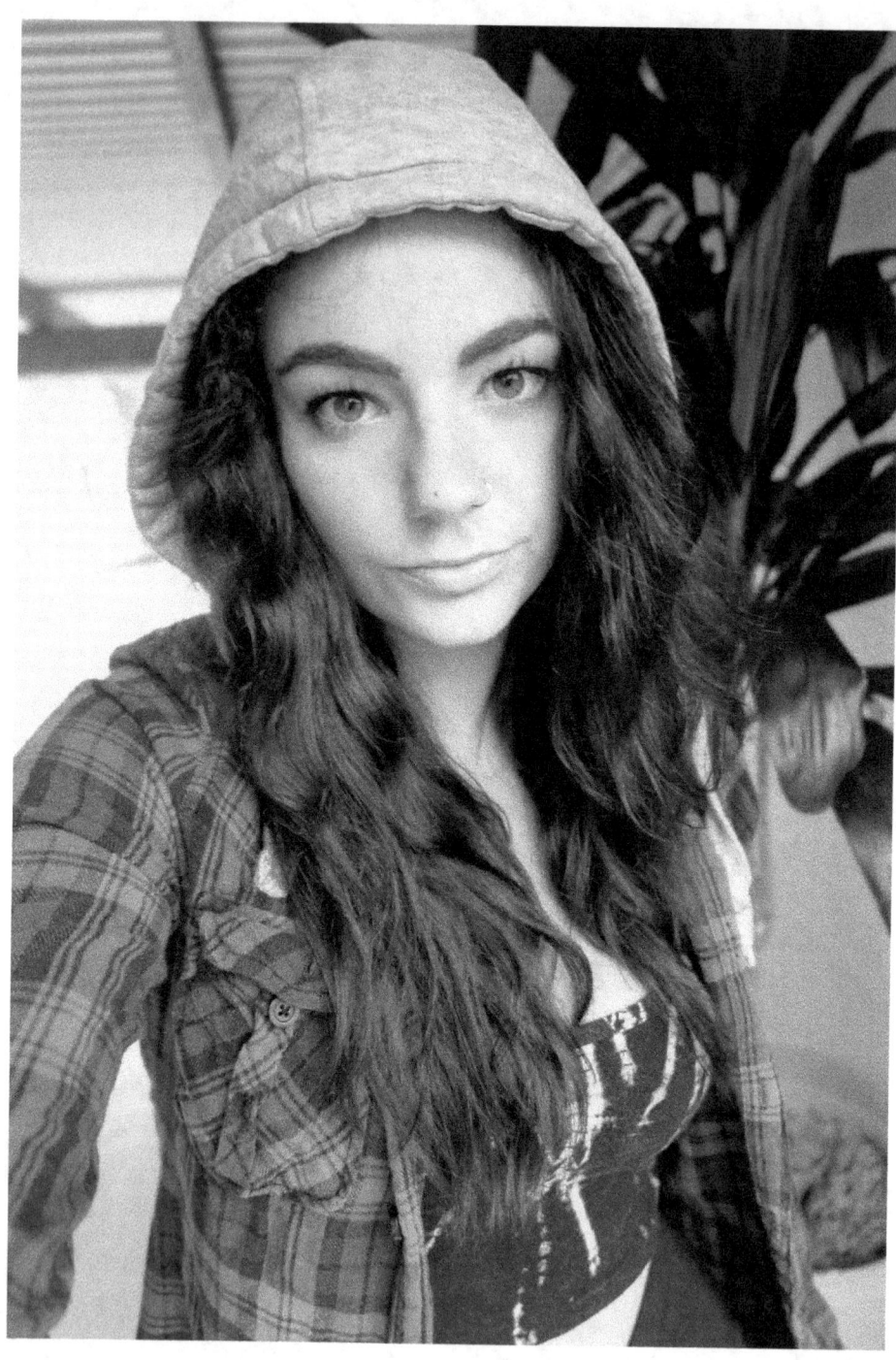

Dear Diary,

I often wonder what level of intimacy people are prepared for when they ask me how I am? I often respond with "I'm okay," just to make it kind of neutral. I rarely say, "I am not okay," to anyone but myself. Yet I hear other people use the phrase all the time. I wonder what they mean. Perhaps I am just gauging what level of empathy to show, or maybe I am actually curious as to how they define the term.

There are different levels of not being okay, and if I'm honest, I haven't been okay for most of my life. Why can't they understand how exhausting that must be for me?

Someone once said to me, "You just need to listen to our point of view because I don't think you understand the carer's side of mental illness ..." I cut them off, saying "Your attitude is so prevalent in society, I know exactly what you are going to say. I've heard it so many times it's practically rammed down my throat! It's seared into my brain! I get it! It's hard for you to know someone who has a mental illness. You want to fucking tell me every time I talk about my mental illness. You want to convince me that it's harder for you to be an observer than a sufferer. How does that make any sense? What other chronic illness gets such stigma?"

I am so sick of hearing how hard *my* disease must be for everyone else but me. Forgive me for being short, but it makes me mad. They all want to be vocal; they all want to be heard, but they don't care to listen to me. The Buddha said, "If you speak, you are only saying what you already know, but if you listen … you might just learn something new." So my patience is running low, and this rant has gone on way too long. The bottom line?

SHUT THE FUCK UP AND LISTEN.

All I want is your presence and trust me, that's enough.

Speaking my Mind Barbie

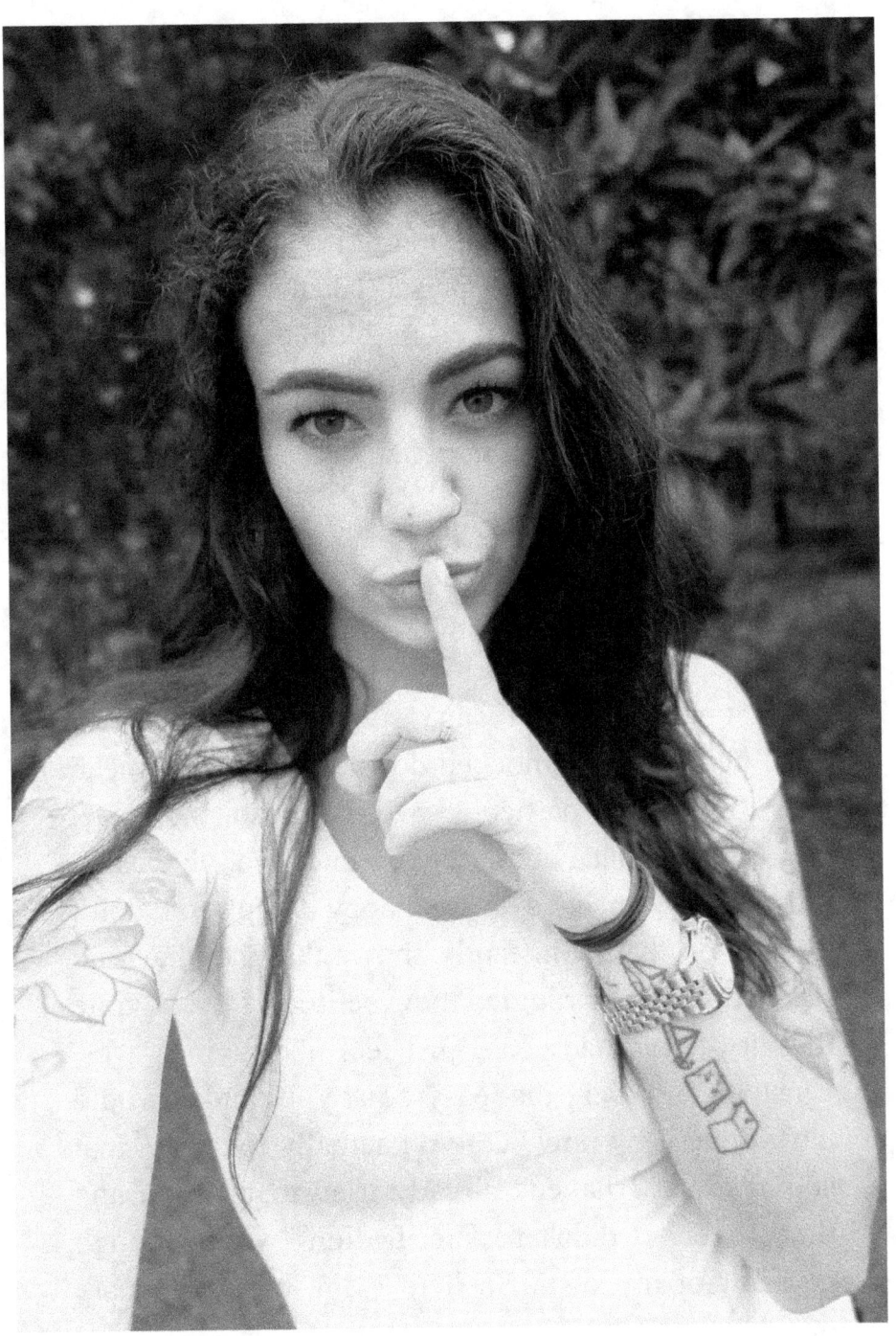

Dear Diary,

People often say to me, "you have so much to be happy about", "find the reasons you have to smile", or "focus on the reasons you have to be happy". It makes me puke in my mouth a little bit. If people think I shouldn't be sad because other people have it worse, is it not the same logic as "I shouldn't be happy since some people have it better?"

I always feel angry and hurt by those comments. It's like they are insulting my intelligence, my awareness and everything I've fought so hard for. It invalidates my struggle. It takes away from how hard I fight every day to stay alive. It's like I am being criticized for trying. Looked down upon because I can't stand up because they don't believe I got knocked down. I know they mean well but those particular words mean the exact opposite to what I am sure they intended. "Focus on the reason you have to be happy" implies I don't already do that. It instantly shows that they have no idea about my struggle; they belittle it every time they try to give advice. I just feel like saying, "Yes Einstein, if it were that easy don't you think I would have done it by now? Do you actually think I'm that stupid? That I haven't already tried that a thousand times over? It didn't fix me. It didn't work, through no fault of my own. So here I am, back to square one."

Sometimes I find the strength to walk away. Sometimes I tell them something along those lines (with varying degrees of profanity). All I ever get as a response is defensiveness. They feel a need to suddenly argue their point, declaring that I'm not doing it properly because it works for them. Well hey, it may work for you, but I'm telling you it didn't work for me, so shut the fuck up.

Sometimes instead of saying, "Just keep a positive mindset," what I really need to hear is, "I know this sucks, I'm here for you". I don't need a lecture or advice. I don't need a cliche. I don't care if you are right or not. My resistance to your suggestions has nothing to do with me saying you're wrong. It is the implications of what your statement implies that stings.

The trouble is not what I have to be happy about, or what I have that makes me smile. That's not the problem. I don't claim to have a lack of total enjoyment. I don't claim that absolutely nothing makes me happy, although sometimes my illness prevents me from doing the things I enjoy. The problem is that I have more to be unhappy about than I do to be happy about. I have more reasons not to smile than I do to smile in the first place. The struggles I face and the mercy of my mind is like an endless cavern. It spills out into every aspect of my life.

Focusing on what I have to be grateful for doesn't really help. It just highlights everything I lack. What I have to be happy about does not get rid of the demons inside me. It just gives them more ammunition to torture me with.

Motivational quotes don't cure my Seasonal Affective Bipolar Disorder, severe Anxiety, PMDD, treatment-resistant Depression, or my Borderline Personality Disorder, nor do they undo years of psychological child abuse. That shit stays with you and will be with me every day for the rest of my life.

I hate the way most people talk to me and about my illnesses (plural) or mental health. Their ignorance infuriates me! Even when someone is knowledgeable, they ask questions just to give advice and not to understand! Oh, that gets under my skin. It's not that I can't see the reasons I have to be happy and the reasons I have to smile. The trouble is those reasons represent less than 1% of my life. That, ladies and gentlemen, is the real issue.

It is not because I choose for it to be so. It is not from a lack of effort on my part. I try as hard as I can to fill my life with things that make me happy. Hundreds of times a day I take a deep breath and say let's appreciate this brief moment of peace, happiness and tranquillity. I treasure every reason I have to smile because I have so many more not to. I hold onto those moments and store them away in a memory bank for reflection on a rainy day.

I hate my illness for taking my smile away. Trust me when I say I don't go down without a fight. But it's never been as simple as putting a smile on my face. What good is a smile if it's hiding a world of pain anyway? I want to feel the smile as it radiates from my heart and soul and shines out on my face, not use it as a tool to please others. I like those real smiles more. Others seem so forced. I wear many smiles in a day. Every day I wake up and put my game face on. I focus on the positive. I practice gratitude. But that does not erase the troubles of the day. It simply gives me the courage to face them.

Gratitude Barbie

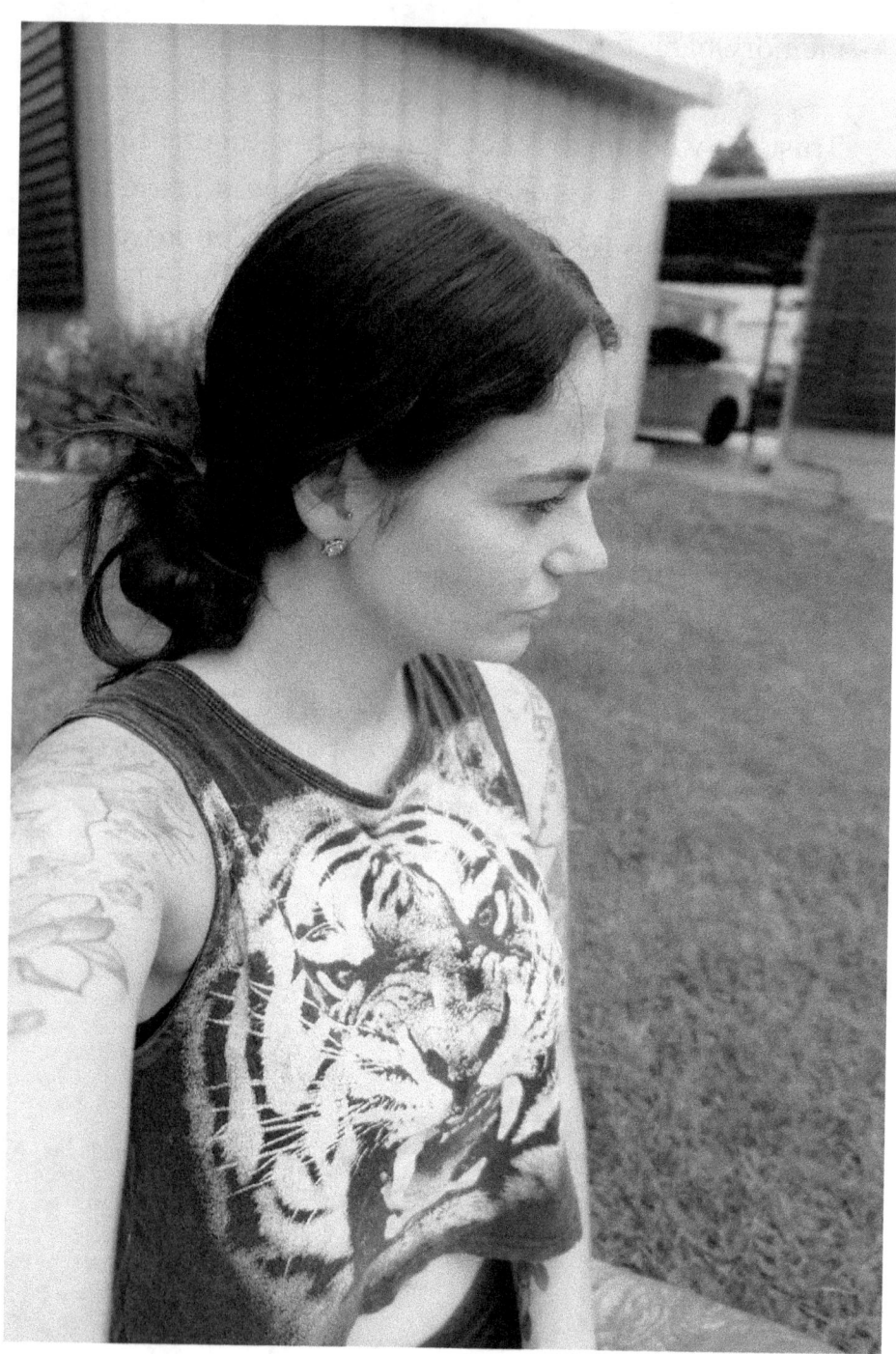

Dear Diary,

My Dad said to me today, "sometimes in life you just have to do things you don't want to do, I do", implying that I chose to avoid doing things I don't want to do.

"I do things I don't want to do every day", I replied.

"Like what?" he asked.

"Every day I force myself to live, even when I really don't want to. That takes all the strength and determination I have. There's not much energy or willpower left after that to force myself to do the rest."

That is the greatest battle anyone will ever face. Forcing yourself to survive when you don't want to live. Not many people know the pain of forcing yourself to be here on this earth and enduring immeasurable pain. How could you when living comes so easy to you? It's not a matter of me choosing to do nothing or avoiding all the things I should be doing because they are too hard. I don't avoid doing things; I try and fail. That is my curse. I will try so hard to lift it. But it's a weight that is too heavy for my shoulders to bear. I am weighed down by it and live in constant fear of it crushing me alive. But somehow, I always survive. By chance? I think not. I work damn hard to keep myself alive!

People love to try to tell me how to live my life. The standard advice is that there is no time for self-pity. "People with depression should be able to just tough it out," they say. They imply we're not strong enough for what's ahead of us, and that we need to get a grip on reality before it's too late. That's crap! And you know what else? They are all wrong when they say people who struggle with mental illness are weak! It takes more courage than any other person in this world has ever exhibited for me just to show up each day. It requires strength beyond belief even though I feel like a shadow of who I used to be.

Warrior Barbie

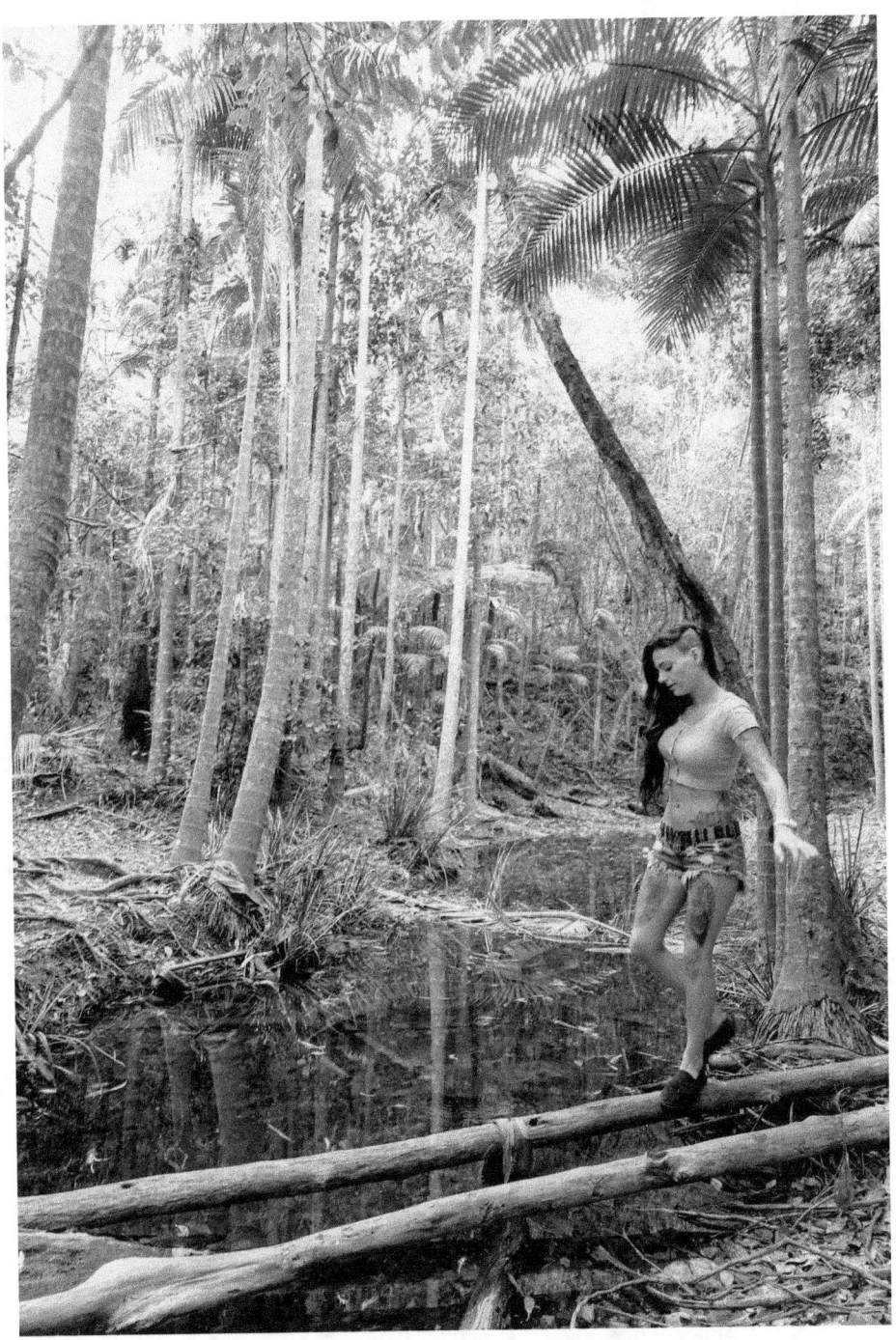

Dear Diary,

There's a primitive survival instinct in all of us. No matter how many times I've tried to kill myself my brain has forced me to survive at all costs even against my own will. I have literally almost drowned in the real ocean more than once, and I always made it back to shore, even when I would have rather sunk below. It's the same reason why today – despite crying many times and being an emotional mess wanting to just give up – I am still here.

I've been told my ego is what makes me sick, seeking help is what keeps me ill and speaking out is what proves all this among many other very ignorant and naive accusations.

I don't doubt that much of what I deal with has a lot to do with me. But don't for a second think I don't know that, because I do and it haunts me every day. But it seems that, in an attempt to explain my illness, it has been misconstrued by many as using it as an excuse.

I've been to the deepest depths of my subconscious, and I've toured the caverns of my soul. I've reflected so much on my life, and my role in everything that has happened around me. Accepting that I have been largely at fault doesn't mean others aren't too.

The more aspects of my illness I explore and

publicise the more excuses people think I'm making and that my real problem is with making excuses.

Mental illnesses, just like ourselves, are so individual and unique there's no right or wrong. It's a lifelong journey to figure it all out. I haven't figured it out, and I don't claim to. I don't mind if no one acknowledges my illness or that they don't congratulate me for all my hard work. I don't expect that of anyone. But what I do expect is respect. To not be talked over the top of, to not be drowned out, to not be discredited, to not be thrown out just because I can't be who society wants me to be.

Everyone else thinks because their life is hard and they just deal with it we should be able to as well. I fantasize so much about getting a "real illness" or being severely injured in some form of freak accident because at least then people would accept my handicap, my pain, my struggles. No one would walk up to someone in a wheelchair and say "You know what? It's your fault you can't walk!"

I didn't choose this life, and I am finding the more I get tired of being what others want me to be, the more faithless I become. I get lost under the surface of society and the bright fake smiles they accept. I know very well what people expect of me, and I have been trying to fulfill their desires for years.

I think the idea that anyone who hasn't suffered

a mental illness are the ones most likely to not believe in its existence is false. In my experience, they are normally the most likely to be open to education on the matter. I think the real judgement comes from within the mental health community. People who suffered some sort of similar ailment think they know everyone's struggle. Sometimes, if someone has experienced some form of depression or anxiety, they think they know what it's like to have Bipolar Disorder.

When talking about this topic, generalising and interchanging the words 'mental health' and 'mental illness' is wrong. Everyone will have some form of mental health issue in their life, just as we all have some form of physical health issue. But that doesn't mean you will have a mental illness. It certainly does not mean you will have a chronic mental illness, just the same as how everyone will get physically sick at some point in their lives, but not everyone will get a chronic illness like diabetes or cancer.

Obviously, those with poor mental health can develop mental illness, just as maintaining poor physical health can lead to more severe physical illness. There are certainly lifestyle risk factors, but there are also genetic predispositions that some people can do nothing about.

As a result, I think there's a huge divide in the mental health community between those who suffer something like depression and anxiety as a result of grief, circumstance or relationship issues. In my experience, more often, people with situational mental health issues find alternative treatments quite effective. They may be able to treat their problems by starting a yoga class, eating healthier, meditating or exercising. They may not need to take medication just as someone with a cold or flu may not need to take antibiotics. Some of them may choose to medicate if severe enough for a while, the same way someone with a knee injury may need to take painkillers. They may just need to rest, make some lifestyle changes and take some time out to heal. But some of us aren't so lucky.

Dr Phil makes a super important point in an interview on Joe Rogan's podcast. He says that a lot of people with depression have extremely valid feelings when you look at what is going on in their life. Medication will only fix a biochemical imbalance or deficiency. If your life is shit, you are going through a separation, your house is burning down, your job sucked and everything is falling apart then you are well within your rights to be depressed. If you didn't feel distressed then you are in serious denial and probably delusional. That then becomes an even bigger problem. There is no point medicating yourself numb because your soul is screaming out that something is seriously wrong in your life. From personal experience, the medication will work for a while and then seem to stop working, but that's because you still are living in a shitty situation and that pain is trying to alert you to something that needs your immediate attention.

I think a lot of people use avoidance and questionable coping mechanisms to trick themselves into believing they are doing fine without proper treatment. I've been there. Maybe that works for some people, but it didn't work for me. The same way just sucking it up and dealing with it didn't work. I know a lot of people think that's the best course of action. If they can do it, why can't I? If I'm not just sucking it up and getting on with my life then I am less of a person, I am weak. But that could not be further from the truth. Sucking it up and dealing with it didn't go so well for me. Unfortunately ignoring my issues only made them worse, as did self-medicating.

I despise the way we lump together all of the 297 unique Mental Illnesses defined in the *DSM (Diagnostic and Statistical Manual of Mental Disorders,* 5th Edition). I try to talk about each of my mental illnesses specifically because they each have their own unique set of challenges, causes and course of treatments. There is a reason they are separated into seven distinct categories, specifically named and given their own pages in the book. They earned their place there by being different from each other. Comparing them would be like opening up a dictionary of all physical ailments that could possibly befall a person and treating them as all the same.

Dr Phil says in his book if you are lying in hospital with a broken leg and the person next to you has just had their leg amputated, people would say that guy has it so much worse than you. But does that make your leg hurt any less? You wouldn't say to someone with a broken leg "stop saying you have a broken leg and it won't be broken" so why do we say that for a broken brain?

To sum it all up, mental illnesses and people suck! People judge, abuse, criticise and accuse others constantly. I ask anyone who starts to judge me, to step into my shoes and walk a mile down the road in the life I am living. I doubt you will get as far as me, but at least you will get a chance to see how strong I really am! You don't need to walk a mile in my shoes, I dare you to live a day in my life. I like to wonder how long it would take someone to start complaining about the massive blisters they would get.

Primitive Barbie

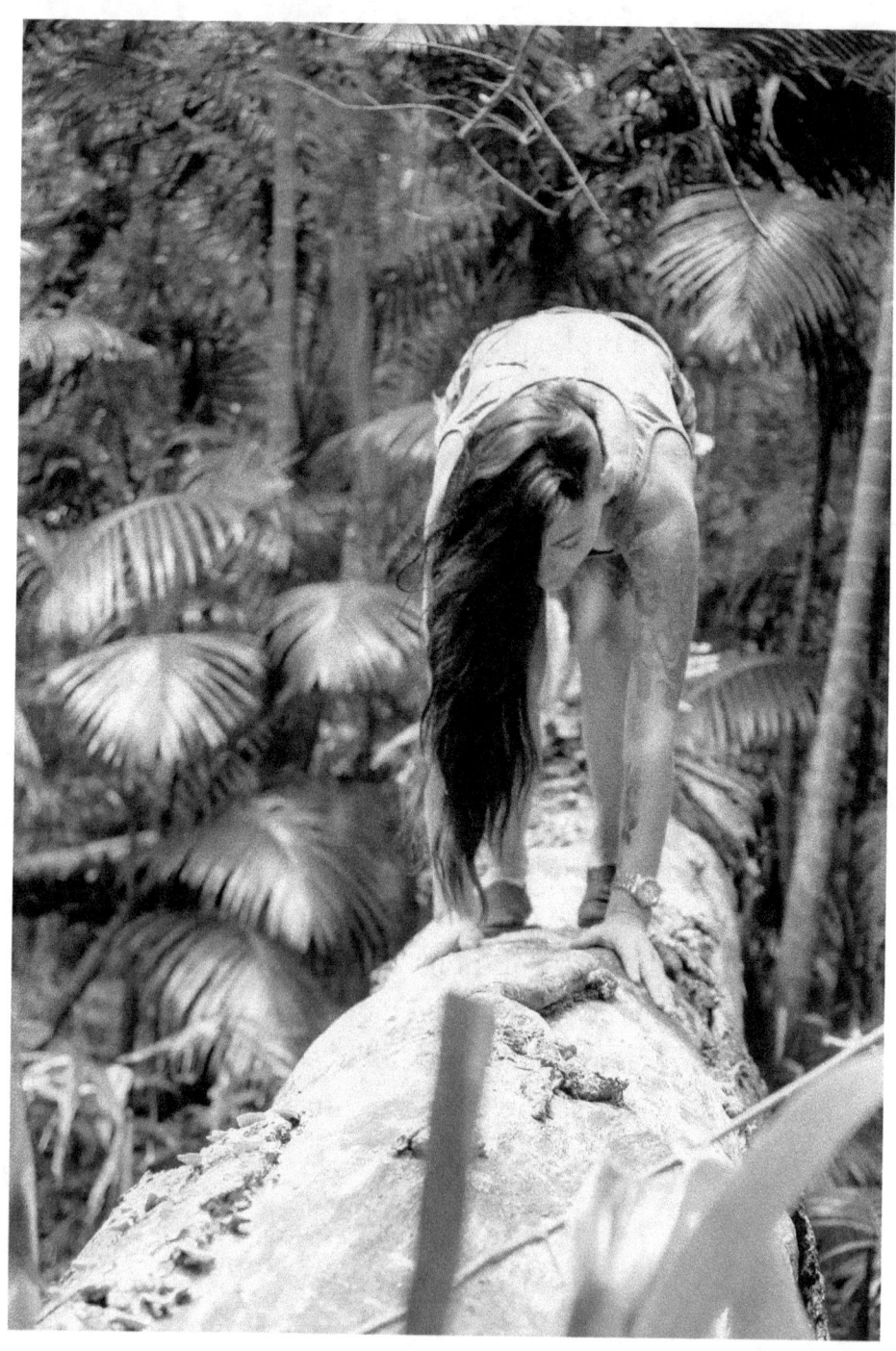

Dear Diary,

We all have those days where we are ready to leave this earth, and the only reason we don't is because the chemist is closed, so we can't get the script we need to drift off into a long eternal sleep. The last thing I want is to cause myself any more pain by doing it in another way. So I make a mental list of the potential ways I can do it and another for the reasons I have to stay alive.

Nothing matters except the only thing I want: an end to my suffering. So I weigh up my options, I cry and try to comfort myself, but nothing sounds more appealing than not being here anymore. Sometimes it's a build up over time, depression or that one last comment from a family member that sends me over the edge. Maybe it's a combination of everything compounded into one dying wish.

I've been wondering for years why I have to live this life. Why is it so hard all the time? All it takes is a few people to tell me that I have chosen this life knowing in my heart I really haven't, to make me question why I even try at all? I must be as useless as they say I am because I don't even dare to take my own life. I am pathetic and weak. Too much of a pussy to pick up the knife and slice through my wrists until they profusely bleed. What a waste of space I am. No wonder everyone else thinks I am a useless human being.

To them, I've either chosen this life or chosen to take my life. But there has never been a choice for me. An ultimatum that my life – and the uneducated opinions of those closest to me – have given me. I can't make my life liveable so why wouldn't I want to die? I wake up every day with a single goal, and I fail miserably every time. I try with all my might to survive, and I live an existence nobody wants to live. And nothing makes me want to give up more than being abandoned by the ones I love.

"It's your fault," they say.

"I's all your fault. You could be like us," they preach, "if you just tried."

They belittle everything I do every day just to function in the desperate way I do. There is nothing more heartbreaking than people around you believing you have destroyed yourself when you're working so hard not to. It's the betrayal of the highest order causing a heartbreak like no other.

My dying declaration is for all the people out there who think they know what they are talking about, who give unsolicited advice on things they claim to understand but have no real knowledge of. It is for all the people who tell me I'm not doing the right things; I'm not trying hard enough to change my situation or blame me for being in this situation in the first place. And for all the people who give advice and claim that I don't listen because if I did, I wouldn't have any problems. Ever think that maybe I have taken your advice – yours and everyone else's in this world – and that it didn't work? Of course you don't, because you simply tell me I must have been doing it wrong or not giving it "my all" because your advice is apparently foolproof! I could be happy, successful and function like the rest of you if I just tried, right? It is for all the people who invalidate me daily, belittling my struggle and undermining how hard I work every single day to overcome it. For those who don't believe I ever had anything to deal with in the first place, and that any troubles I may face are of my own creation. For those people who insult me in the most significant way possible, by doubting my will to be well. And for those accusing me of wanting to be like this, like I get some sick satisfaction from it. Tell me … what do I gain from being like this? Why would I make everything a thousand times harder than it should be?

"Well …" they respond, "if you were trying at all you would be able to turn your situation around and succeed like the rest of us." I am sick of people reading these success stories and tell-all books only to come to the conclusion that overcoming hardship can be condensed into one chapter. My autobiography will have to be an entire series! There is no way this struggle can be squished into one volume. I am sure it would get repetitive, but that is the nature of my existence. I wake up to the same shit each day and go to bed with the same demons every night. It is not one great battle and subsequent story of victory to be told for generations to come. It is a string of tiny fights that will be forgotten.

I want people to know that I turn my situation around every second of every day. To them, if I was, I would be working, earning money, supporting myself, being sociable and happy. Not every situation can be turned around to those extremes. Just because my glass is always half full, doesn't mean I'm not topping it up. Each day it begins empty, and I use every bit of strength to add what little I have at my disposal to it. But that will never be enough for you. Hell, it's never enough for me! I yearn to drink from a glass that's full, but for some reason, my glass is full of holes, and I patch them up every day. I am aboard a leaky vessel with rats burrowing holes into my hull. There is always more. I spend the majority of my time trying to find them (the problem) and patch them up (working out a solution).

I have turned a lot around in my lifetime. Today I've convinced myself not to end it all half a dozen times. I've turned around my will to die and tried to find my will to live. But to you, I've just spent the day mostly in bed and soaking in the bath. To you, I have done nothing to help myself. I also did my laundry today, something I haven't been able to do in a month. I try as hard as I can to fight the war inside my head, and until I have conquered the battles of today, then I have no chance at living.

I am just as frustrated as you – if not more – that I am in the same place I have been before. I am fighting a war I just can't seem to win, and as each day goes by, I realise how long this war really could go on for. But regardless of whether you have mental health issues or not, yours will never be the same as mine or another's. Just because you could cure yours with mind over matter or a simple pill, doesn't mean I'm not trying hard enough when numerous medications later still haven't "cured" me. Maybe they never will. Don't imply another isn't trying hard enough because they keep saying nothing is working. Maybe it's really not. That's not me making excuses, that's me asking for help.

Don't ever question how helpless, hopeless and disheartened I feel every second of every day. I did not choose this life, but I am strong enough to live it. So don't you dare make me feel weak for living a life you don't even take the time to understand. I don't claim I know everything about mental illness, mine or yours. I am always learning, so don't shut your mind off, or be naïve enough to think you have the solution to complex problems even a team of professionals can't figure out. If it was as simple as you say it is … then I wouldn't still be living in hell.

Every day I choose to fight. When I look at myself in the mirror, I see all my flaws. I see everything I am facing and everything I am forced to overcome. I don't see the lie I tell myself; the story I try to convince myself of every day. "I am strong," I say. "You can do this, you will do this, there has to be a way, and you will find it. I know it will take time, but you have to be close, look at how far you have come!"

That is the attitude I try to live by, it's the only thing keeping me alive. That doesn't mean I am not overwhelmed by the struggle I face. The gravity of my situation threatens to tear me down, but I stand tall in the face of it all. Doesn't that count for something? I wish it did, but it's not enough. Even though there are a few who understand my pain and believe it is real, society won't see it that way. "Who cares what society thinks!" I scream, but their judgement is unshakeable. I see it in myself. It's not society I am letting down, it's me. It's the person that no matter how hard I try I just can't be.

I look at myself and see what they see. "You look fine, why can't you just get on with it and live your life?" I look in the mirror, and I think to myself, *this isn't you.* I don't buy it. Not the fake confident together version of yourself you try to be nor the weak, pathetic incapable excuse of yourself you have become. Neither one is me, I never quite feel like me. I don't know who I am or who I have become, but I am haunted by the person I am, it's not somebody anyone wants to be. I don't want to destroy myself, but I'm afraid to push myself because I fail so much.

I am told constantly about how much potential I have and I don't doubt it. "But don't you see?" I beg. "I see everything you see in me. But think how frustrating it must be to watch myself waste away, held back, suffocated and strangled in this way. You ask me if I want more for myself. Every single day I try but no matter how hard I try my best isn't good enough. Don't you see how heartbreaking that must be for me? But you can't see what holds me back, so you assume I choose to waste my days and "potential" away. A waste maybe, but not because I want it to be that way."

Waste of Space Barbie

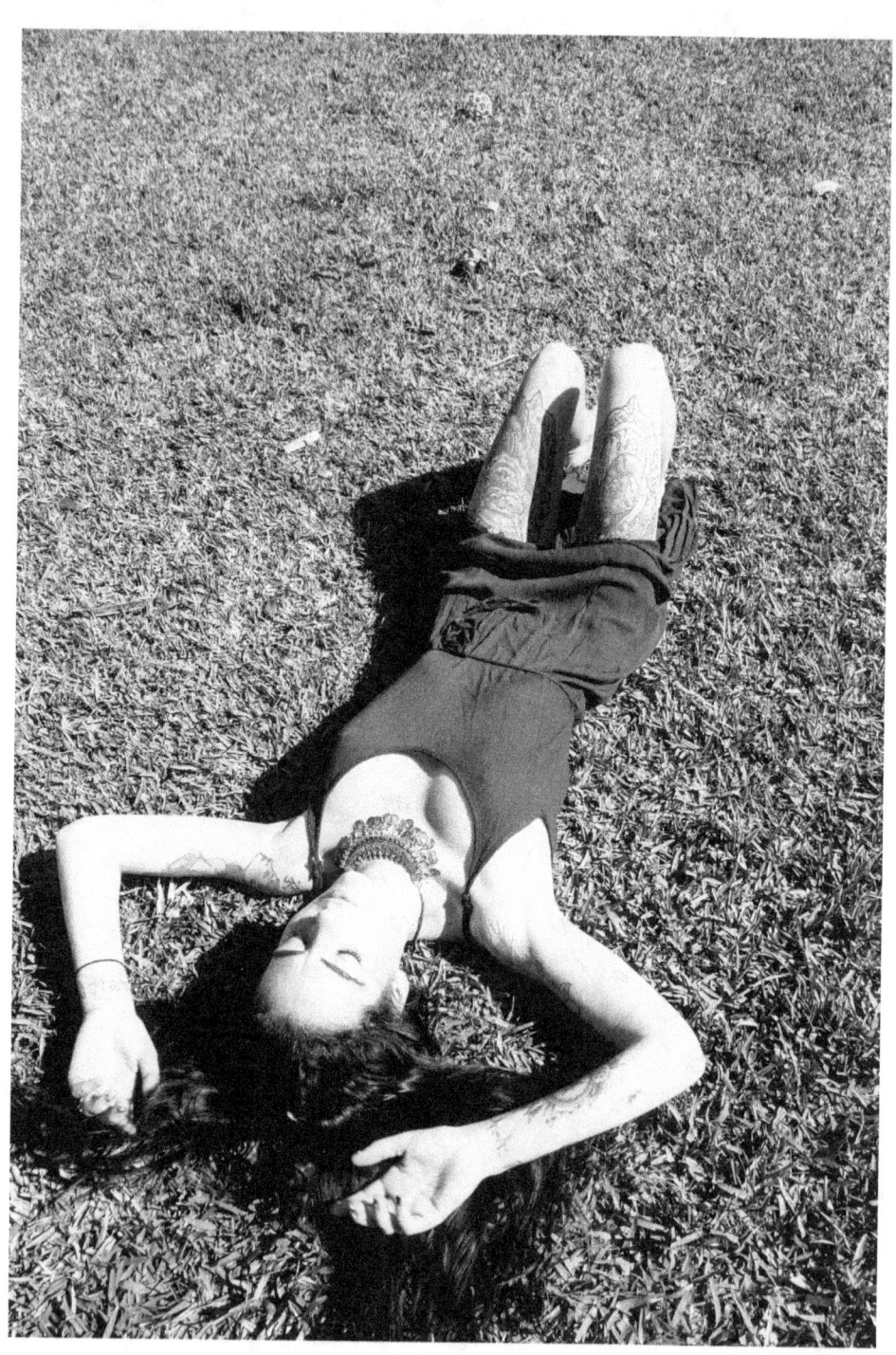

Dear Diary,

I let it all out in my psychology session the other day. I was dreading it all morning. I was mentally preparing myself for what I was about to do. Normally I get nothing out of those visits that I don't already know. Why do I continue to go? It just seems to be the thing to do. Doctors won't prescribe me medication unless I go. The government won't assist me unless I go. No one will take me seriously unless I go. Therapy is meant to solve all of my problems. I play along. It's all part of the game. I mainly go there to celebrate my week's successes and to whine about my failures. There aren't too many of them because failure is not an option. At least as far as the rest of the world is concerned. Deep down I already feel like a failure and even when I succeed it makes me feel terrible for even struggling to do things in the first place.

Normally I just jump straight into it. I found it hard to start and get it all off my chest today. I've seen this woman almost every week for about a year now. I think yesterday was the first day I spoke about something real. It was like admitting my greatest secret. She was so surprised she doubted it could be true. No one knows. I've become so good at hiding it. The only problem with hiding it is not that the truth will come out eventually. I've prevented myself from solving the problem. I think that just made it so much worse. So today we sat down to map out the particulars of my sense of self and lack of self-worth. I think she began to understand. She gave me a large sheet of paper and encouraged me to write it all down. Everything I wanted to put down seemed like the truth and a lie. I have spent a lifetime convincing myself I am who I want to be and hiding who I am. I am even confused about where one begins and the other ends. They have become so intertwined that I can feel them knotted up in my stomach. She told me that having Borderline Personality Disorder amplifies your emotions. Even I struggled to put words to it. Self-hate, self-loathing, incredible inadequacy and worthlessness don't even begin to describe how I feel about myself.

I have felt so confused and vulnerable since my psychiatrist visit on Monday. I let myself experience who I was without hiding it, covering it up, pushing it aside or filing it away. It has been an uncomfortable three days. Facing it was difficult, it still is. It's a lump in my throat that I haven't been able to swallow. Tears have been welling in my eyes. My heart is being torn out of my body. I am being eaten from the inside out.

My mind has been dwelling on it as I always do. I have had to figure out what it is, why, when, where and how it got there. I've also struggled a lifetime with the most important question. How do I fix it? How do I make it go away? I've temporarily suppressed it, but it is still there. Maybe I am not depressed for seventy percent of the year. Maybe the only time I ever feel good about myself is when I am manic. Maybe even my "normal" is dark.

After today's session, I struggled. I'm not sure what is the truth and what is a lie. It is a grey area I need to figure out. "Fake it till you make it" hasn't worked out so well for me. "How do I fix it?" is still running through my mind. I hear crickets in the distance. A part of me does feel relieved. I have shared that burden, and at least one person is on my side. Her job is to help me, and I have finally admitted that is what I need the most. Today has been such a relief. I feel like I have been honest for the first time in my life.

It's hard to admit that you have a problem, and even harder when you feel like there is no one who understands your pain. In today's society it seems as if everyone is struggling in some way, which does make things easier. I'm not alone in this battle, though sometimes it still feels that way.

Real Barbie

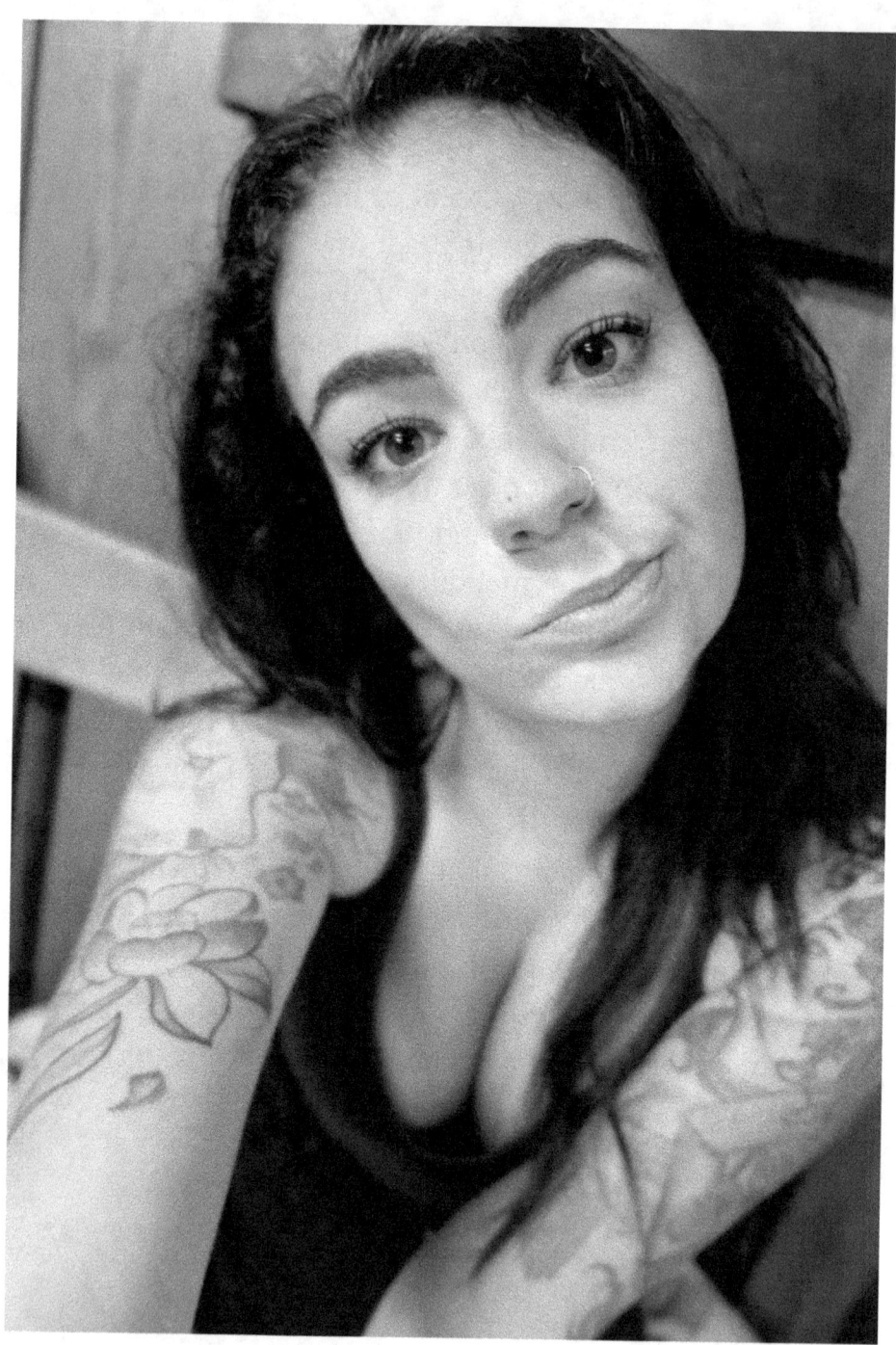

Dear Diary,

I never thought of myself as an actress. Not until I realised I have been acting every single day of my life. I do it so naturally I don't even realise that I'm doing it now. Sometimes I can't even tell the difference between what is the real me and what is an act. I am pretty good at hiding what I am really feeling. But at some point, the cracks begin to show.

Pretending to be okay as my life fell apart around me became quite exhausting after a while. Eventually I had to admit I wasn't. I had to admit the real reason my life was in turmoil, because otherwise people would have kept on accusing me of deliberately destroying my life. Why would anyone want to do that?

Since I've been speaking openly and honestly about my mental health, people seem to think I do it for attention. That I "play" mentally ill. An oscar worthy performance they assure. But they are not fooled and every single one of them wants to be the one to uncover the truth! They are all like journalists investigating an expose. "You're not mentally ill! You're just fucked up!" They are like a bunch of internet sleuths determined to reveal a deep-rooted conspiracy theory.

People often ask me, "What happened to you? Why did the person we love start suddenly acting like this?" The truth is that what they had seen before this was all an act. The whole time I had been covering up a dark secret, hiding behind fake smiles, pretending to be happy and have my shit together when I didn't. I had the energy to do it then, but like a car, I quickly depreciated in value and my engine no longer ran so well. Things got so bad there was no way of hiding it. So I decided to get real. I had to if I had any chance of helping myself. I had to admit something was wrong first!

I don't make excuses. Even though I am often accused of making them. I offer my story to the ones around me as an explanation; an attempt to connect with others through understanding and education. Unfortunately I am often distanced by ignorance and stigmatisation.

I am truly alone. Maybe not physically, but it has become clear that this is a journey I have to undertake on my own. I don't want to. I would give anything for it not to be so. But I don't have a choice. No one is there for me. Despite how hard I try to reach out to them. Perhaps I don't try as hard as I think. It has begun to hurt too much. I am just going to stop trying. At first, it was extremely disheartening and traumatic to be ignored and dismissed. But looking back now it was the most important part of my recovery. It was only when they were gone that I began to rely on myself. (Like I had been doing the whole time anyway.) When I stopped wasting my energy swimming towards people who retreated from me, reaching out to people who didn't want to be reached I found myself making progress. I had to acknowledge that no one else was going to save me. So I was faced with the tough choice: to give up or to rescue myself. I've always been a resilient, stubborn bitch. Just ask my father. Daddy didn't raise a quitter. He may have raised an emotionally unstable train wreck, but he certainly did not raise a quitter. So I summoned my inner warrior, suited up and prepared myself for battle. I armed myself with the tools I needed to win this war.

I didn't ask to be cast in this role. I was thrust into it. If I could choose a role to play, I would play the dedicated, successful, goal driven, enthusiastic, life loving girl that I used to be. I liked playing her. I mourned her loss for years. I still *do* to this day. I refused to let her go, but she was taken for me. It took years to accept that I wasn't her anymore. I live in hope I might be her again someday, but for now, I am someone different. I am mentally ill. A plot twist I would never have written for myself.

People criticise me for saying that. They say, "If you keep telling yourself you are mentally ill, you will become mentally ill."

Ha-ha. "But I do have mental illnesses." That is a fact, not a fabrication of my own creation. I can't just will it away. I've tried that. It didn't work for me.

If I don't acknowledge them or neglect to tend to them, I am neglecting myself.

I often talk about what I face because not many people understand that. I describe the feelings, sensations, thoughts, symptoms and how it affects my life. I lay it out the way I experience it. But for every observation I make about myself and my life I am working ten times harder to overcome it. Every thought I have is carefully screened for negative thinking styles and adjusted accordingly.

I fight every day to overcome the obstacles I face. Just because I don't detail the lengths I go to just to counter every negative aspect of my illness doesn't mean I don't work damn hard to deal with this shit every day! Just because I talk about the hurdles I have to overcome doesn't mean I don't plan to overcome them.

I have a goal, direction, determination and a ferocious fight within me! I don't wake up thinking, *how can I be mentally ill today?* I wake up thinking, *what is affecting me today and how can I overcome it? How can I do all the things I have to do, while managing my illness? How can I have the best day possible?*

When I say, "this is what I experienced today, this is what I observed", what I really mean is, "this is what I had to overcome today."

Stigmatisation is ripe in our society, and that is because most people have a severe lack of understanding. I believe that ignorant attitudes towards mental illness and those of us that suffer stems from a lack of comprehension rather than a lack of compassion.

Awareness isn't about this word 'stigma'. It shouldn't be about the people who reject mental illness and deny its legitimacy or the people who ignore our struggles. Mental health awareness should be about us, about everyone and what we experience. How do we do that? People need to be educated to grasp the essence of what it means to be mentally ill before they can be empathetic towards our plight.

Education doesn't always happen in the classroom or a formal setting. Education happens every day in life. We are constantly learning. Our subconscious is being programmed by everything we see, hear, smell, touch and taste. We are being tutored every waking hour of our lives without realising it. As humans we are designed to assess the world around us and create a blueprint for our default behaviours based on external stimuli. Our main motives for our actions are physical survival and acceptance.

I believe mental health should be spoken about openly and honestly, so I lead by example. I believe in being the change I want to see in the world. We can all play our part in changing the face of mental health. I give a creative take on living with mental illness in the hopes of not only inspiring others to keep fighting, but also to encourage everyone else to talk about mental health too. I tell my story and reveal myself in a raw and honest way to encourage others to do the same.

Actress Barbie

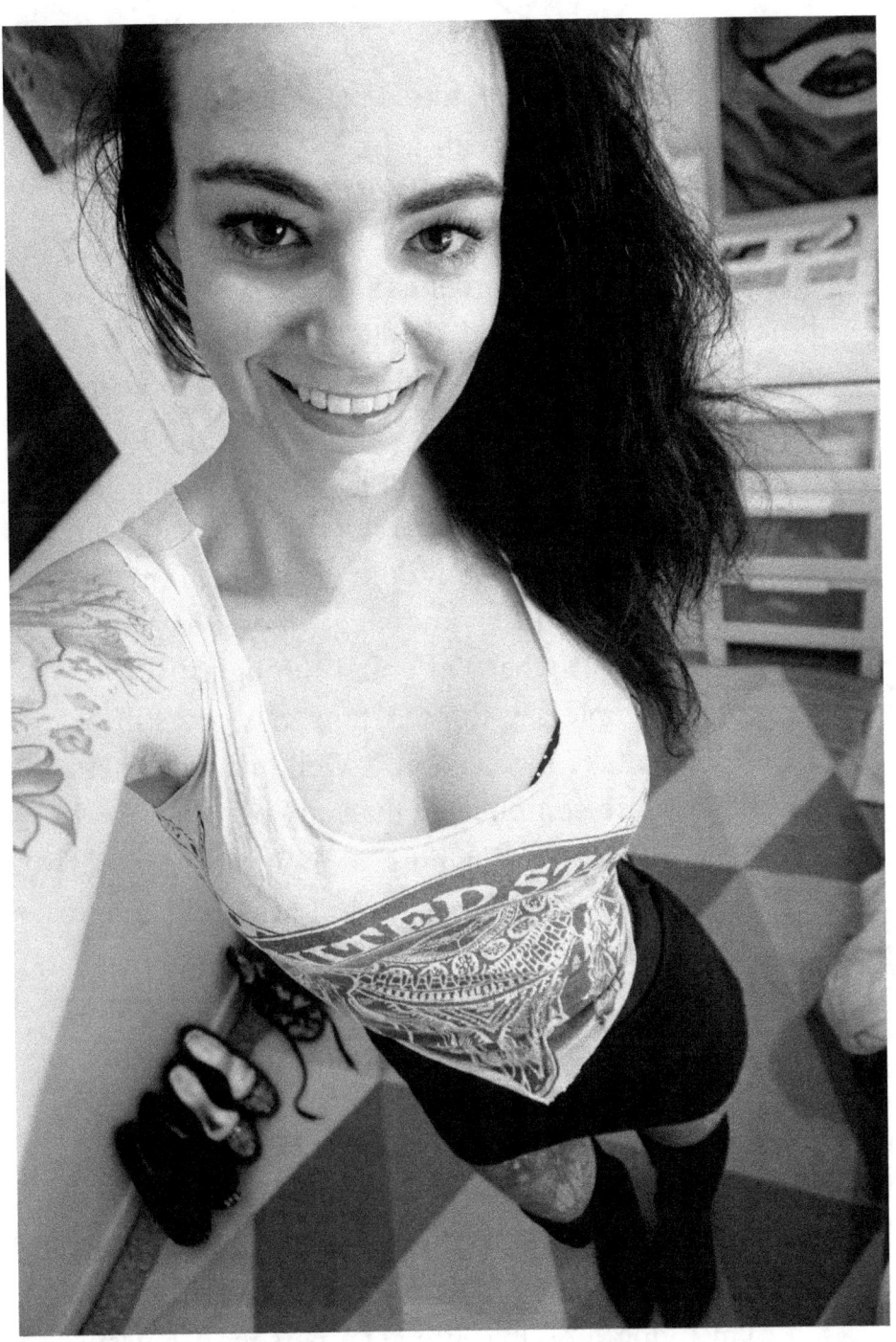

Dear Diary,

Sometimes I feel like I am gasping for air. Struggling to breathe with a huge heavy weight on my chest or in my head. Each day I walk around feeling like I'm about to internally combust, choking back the lump in my throat as I swallow my fears. I think it's my hopes and dreams that I struggle to swallow the most. They are just too big and force me to choke.

I get sick of screaming for help. Everyone just looks at me, confused wondering why I am struggling when they are all doing just fine. It makes me feel angry, just knowing they have no comprehension of what I'm going through. It drives me *insane*! People say to me, "how can you still be unwell if you take medication?" Well, mental illness is so much more complicated than any pill.

It is difficult to diagnose a brain disorder and near impossible to understand it. I was told today that to get the help I need; I have to stop being strong. I was always taught to be strong. ("Stay strong, keep going! Get your shit together girl!" everyone preaches.) I was told to stop putting so much effort into being a functioning individual and let the world or organisations in question know the real struggles I face. It goes against every bone in my body. It isn't in my nature to do that.

I'm living a double life. The persona I put out

in the world and how I feel inside are vastly different. All I achieve is making the people around me feel more comfortable while I rot away in hell. The internal daily struggle is a tug of war between how I want to be perceived and who I really am. I pretend everything is fine, and as a result, people assume I am fine. And sometimes I'd rather not tell anyone because I have learnt over the last few years that people can be evil. The more you let them know about you, the more ammunition they have to use against you. Sometimes I wish I had never told anyone anything about myself. I know there are people in this world who will use my truth against me. It's been done before. I expect that type of betrayal now.

I stop and think for a second when I want to share a moment of weakness with someone. I pause because I know what nasty people could do with that information. It has made me feel like there is no one I can trust. The only thing that makes me think twice about that resolve is my *Instagram* account. I have seen how owning my story and loving myself through that process is the bravest thing that I will ever do.

I am always asked how I find the words to describe what's going on in my mind. The truth is I've always had them. That's what keeps me posting and encourages me to keep sharing. I know I am one of the few with that ability. I consider it my duty to show the world what we deal with every day. Even if I have to be the sacrificial lamb being led to the slaughter. I know it's worth it for the greater good. I want people to know my struggle is real and I want those who struggle to know that they are not alone.

Advocate Barbie

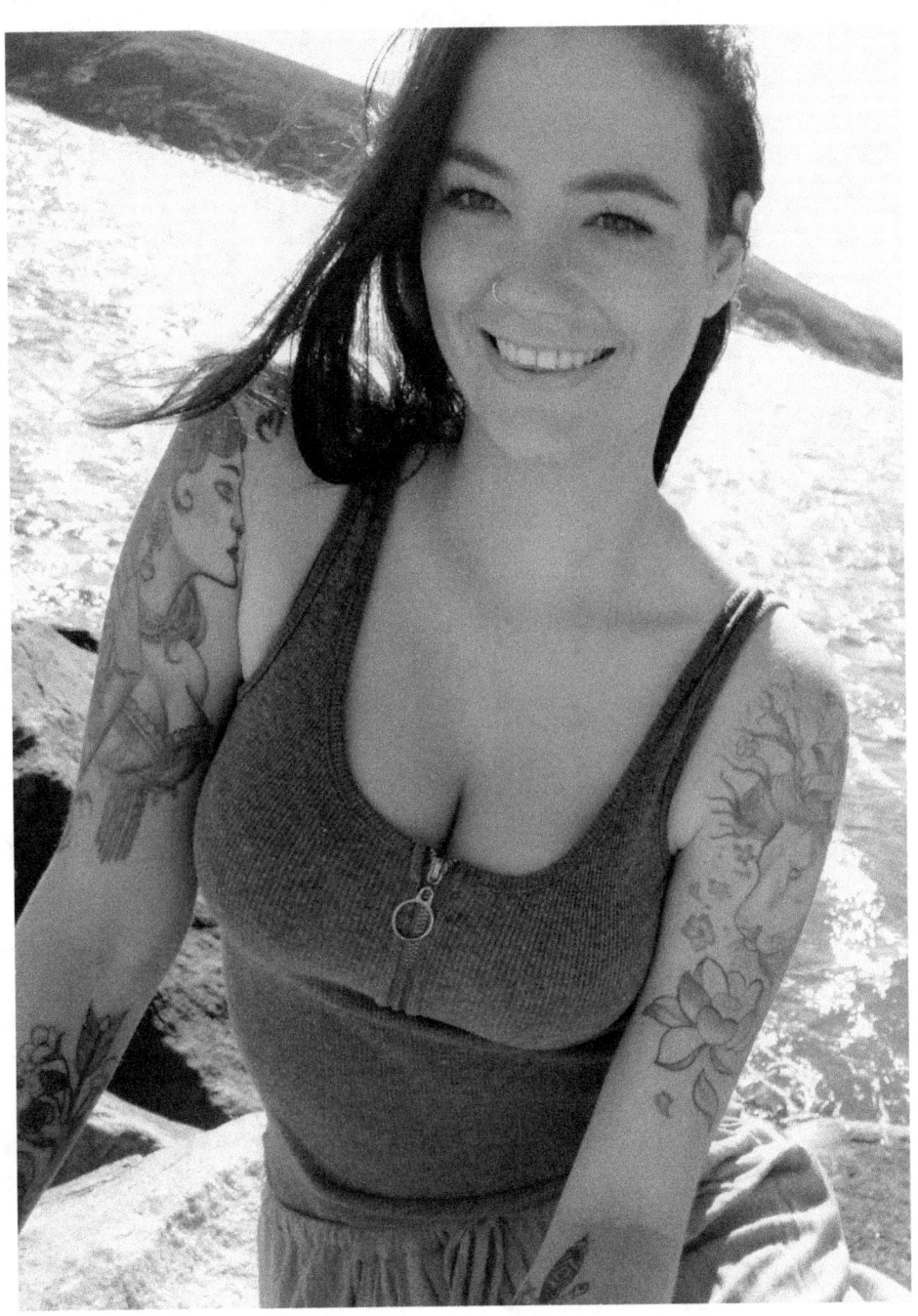

If you can't get out of the seas of mental illness, then you might as well learn to swim

Bipolar Barbie

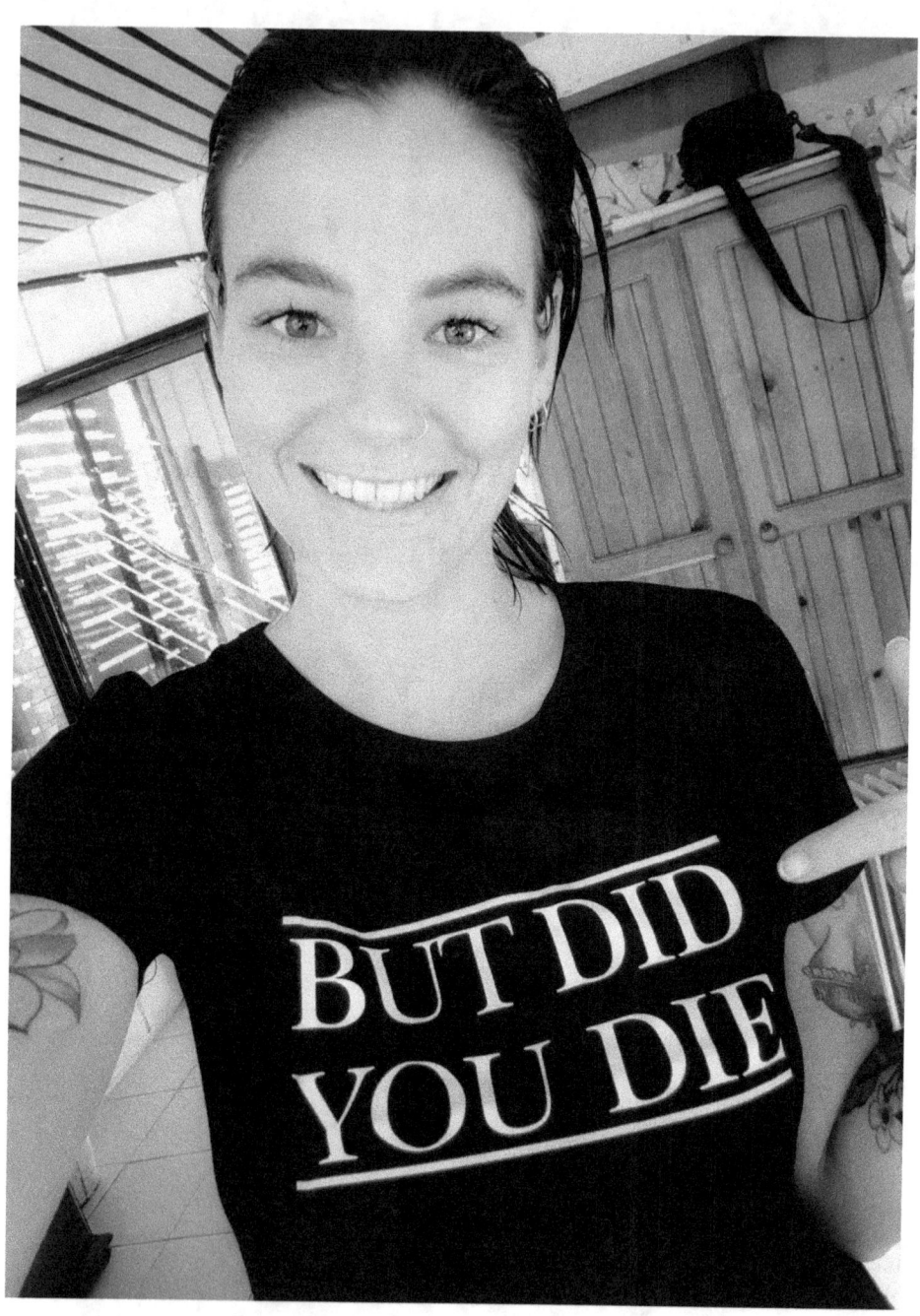

Dear Diary,

For a while now, I haven't had the luxury of standing. I haven't been able to rest or relax. I am always treading water. Even when I look like I'm doing okay, I am fearful that at any moment I could sink below the water to the bottom of the deep dark ocean.

It reminds me of being a Surf Lifesaver, and all those years I spent at the beach when I was a kid. That terrifying feeling of being at the mercy of the sea. Sometimes it's like being caught in a wave that swallows you up before forcefully spitting you out. Or like being stuck in the spin cycle of a washing machine. It disorientates you and holds you under until you are desperate for air. Your life doesn't flash before your eyes, but the very real possibility of dying right now, on this day, does. There's a sense of fear and shock, but also a startling stillness and calm.

It's when the tumbling motion of the wave stops, that you find yourself swimming with all your might. It's like automatically your body seizes the opportunity to save itself before you even know what's happening. For a brief moment, I am relieved and excited that I am finally getting somewhere. I am so desperate for air at this point, I know if I don't break through the surface soon, I will surely suffocate. So, I eagerly seize the chance to save myself.

But that excitement and sense of opportunity rapidly vanish the moment my hands touch the sand on the ocean floor. The moment I realized I had been frantically swimming in the wrong direction. You quickly re-orientate yourself, so you can propel to the surface as soon as possible. Your lungs are now burning. Screaming for air. But unfortunately, the eight-to-twelve second window between that wave and the next has passed. You're going to break through the surface just as it hits. Let's hope you get enough air in to survive the next spin cycle!

Some days, you might get lucky and there may be more time in-between each wave. Other days, there may only be seven waves in a set and on others still, there may be upwards of fifteen. Sometimes, there may be a minute to get back to shore before the next set hits. Some days, you might make it. Some days, you might not.

Some days are calm, but even on those days, I am still way out of my depth. It's always just a matter of time before the next episode hits. I am at the mercy of the tide. The rotation of the moon as it orbits the earth. I am floating, nearly drowning, always treading water. I am desperate. Tired of these endless seas. I lost direction long ago and no matter how hard I try to find it, even when I grasp it, in an instant it disappears again.

I can't seem to find my way back home. I am

disorientated. An ocean explorer without a compass. My world has been turned upside down and I am Captain Jack Sparrow running back and forth on a pirate ship from starboard to port side rocking the boat until it flips. I travel to the ends of the earth waiting for the sun to set until I realise sundown is the rise of the world's end. The end is the beginning and upside down is the right way up. What dangers await me in the seas of hell?

    I am cold and weary of this tiresome fight. An endless plight that seems to have no end. Stretching as far as the ocean itself, no one knows how deep these seas really are. Just when you think you have reached the bottom it falls away beneath your feet and you are once again sinking into the abyss. I feel trapped at the mercy of each storm that rages on overhead. Clear blue skies give me a passing minute to catch my breath, but there is no time to feel relieved. Because I have come to know that at any minute the tides will turn and I will be sent back to the unknown. Yet this place is all I have ever known, so I wonder if the true unknown lies up ahead? The place I am constantly searching for but may never find. How can I be sure it even exists? It seems like a myth.

    I try to remember what it was like to live on the land. With my feet firmly planted on the ground. Not a care in the world, I wandered this earth never fearing the dirt vanishing beneath my feet. Yet here I am with no place to stand wondering what I ever stood for. The very air I breathe tastes bitter. Maybe it's the salt water so generously lapping against my lips that makes the air taste so crisp. I fear each breath like it contains a contagion more dangerous than anyone has ever seen. To me, it tastes like death. But I do not fear death, in fact I worship it. I fantasize about the ways I will come upon my end. I wish for it every day. I detest breathing because with it comes the burden of life. My life, the very thing I despise.

    I am alone, afraid and floating in the great unknown. I am lost somewhere in the seas of mental illness. When will I find my way back home?

Disorientated Barbie

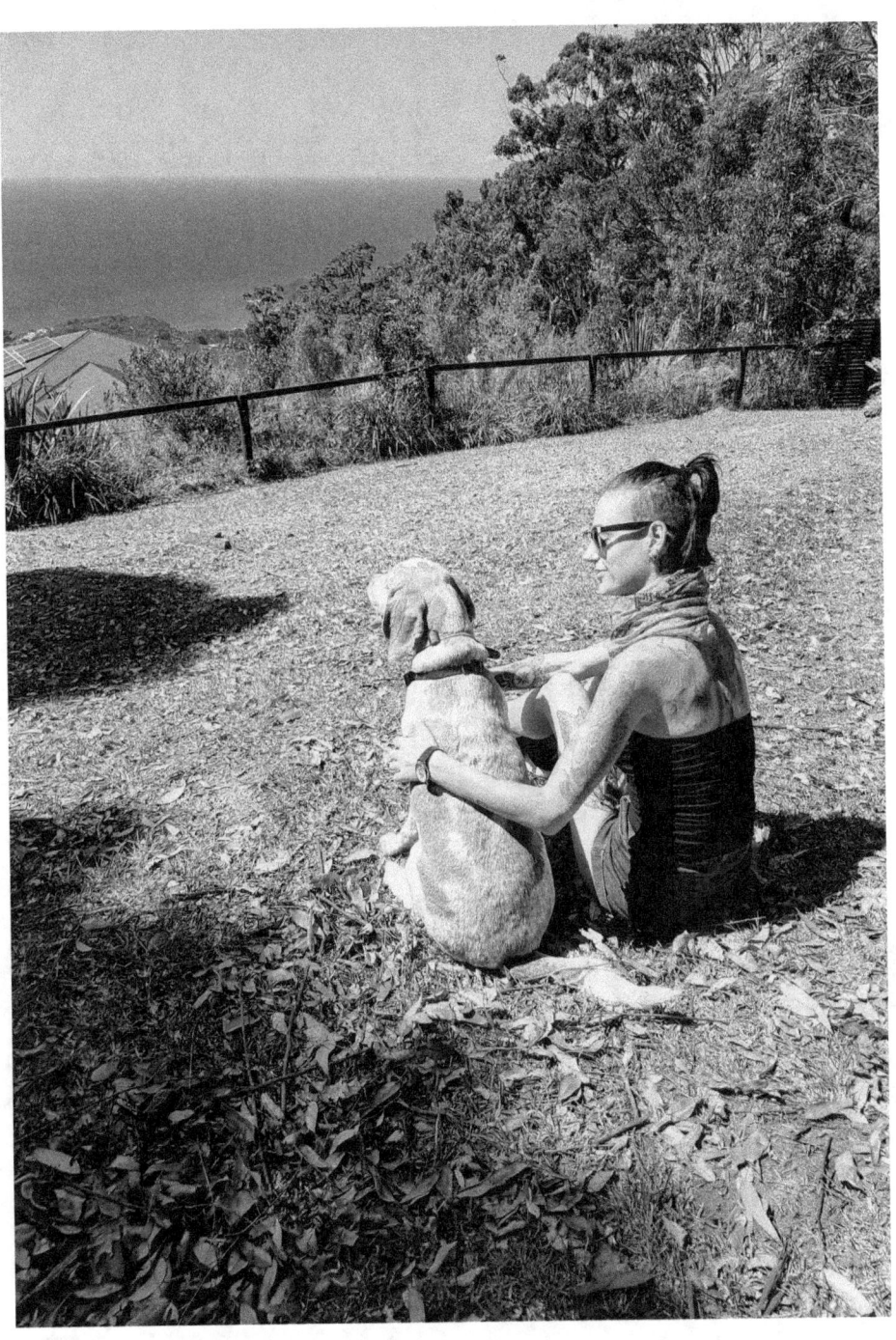

Dear Diary,

I used to think I knew who I was. Until I realised I had no freaking idea. Then I felt like a naïve idiot for ever being arrogant enough to believe I ever did. I don't know if I will ever truly know myself. Although I seem to have figured some of it out over the past few years. Sometimes you really do have to destroy yourself to find yourself. You have to strip away a lifetime of conditioning and people telling you who you are so that you can finally see yourself for who you *really* are or who you always were.

Trust me though. It's pretty damn hard to shake a lifetime of negative criticism and conditioning. Especially from your parents. I don't know how people can be surprised that kids can grow into adults thinking they are a piece of shit because they were told every day that's what they were. People are weird. I don't know why we are so stubborn and unwavering in our personal beliefs that we resist change.

I have come to learn that we change with every interaction we have. Every second of our lives we are evolving, being moulded and shaped by the stimuli we are exposed to. For better or worse. Sometimes more than others. So I think the moment you decide you know who you are is the moment you become a stranger to yourself. I thought I knew who I was until suddenly I didn't feel like that person anymore. Everything I had been capable of, I suddenly wasn't. Everything I used to find easy was suddenly hard. My world was turned upside down like I'd been picked up and dropped off in Topsy Turvy town. Whatever the hell that is! It's certainly a place in hell though. Maybe a suburb on the outskirts of Satan's evil city. All I know is that I did travel to the ends of the earth. I had to decipher what was really me and what was my illness. I question that every second of every day. I am well aware of all that I am not anymore, the people around me have made sure of that. But because of all that I had lost, I felt like I was nothing. It didn't occur to me at first that I had gained anything. After all, mental illness is the most cunning thief I've ever heard of. If only I could train it to rob a bank ... Sure, I wish all of this had never happened to me because living with it feels like a burden too painful to carry. But there is no denying it has shaped me into the person I am today.

It has been a trek through the jungle. But the worst part was feeling like I was isolated and shipwrecked on an island. I spent years signalling for help but one saw the smoke.

Friends keep telling me that I can call them if I want to talk about it. But the fact is, there's nothing to talk about. That's how I know it's biological. I feel shit. Full stop. There's no more to it than that. If you can't make it better, then talking about it is going to make it worse. So please don't try to make me feel better with your words. I've already tried, and they will be merely patronising.

I squirm away from human interaction. Please let me hate myself in solitude. All you will do is make me feel worse for not being able to love myself the way I desperately want to. I'd even settle for just liking myself right now. A good day to me is one where I don't want to kill myself. It's sad how that's my only measure of a good day. It's laughable how few and far between they are.

Distraction is key. I watched a movie when I came home. It has put me in a better mood. I got a chance to disassociate to a better place. I enjoyed the chance to get immersed in another world. Isn't that what we all want? Another life? One without the burdens of our hateful mind? Hell, I'd even settle for a world where people understood my struggle, where I wasn't constantly criticised and made to feel like I'm not doing a good enough job. I'm doing the best I can yet I am constantly told it's not enough. What do you do when our best isn't good enough? Most people would answer "give up". Yet in life that's frowned upon. I wish just someone would pat me on the shoulder and say "hey, you're doing your best, I'm sorry it's not good enough" and hold me while I silently reflect about how hopeless I feel. It wouldn't fix my problems. But it would be enough to know I wasn't alone.

Sigh

Robinson Crusoe Barbie

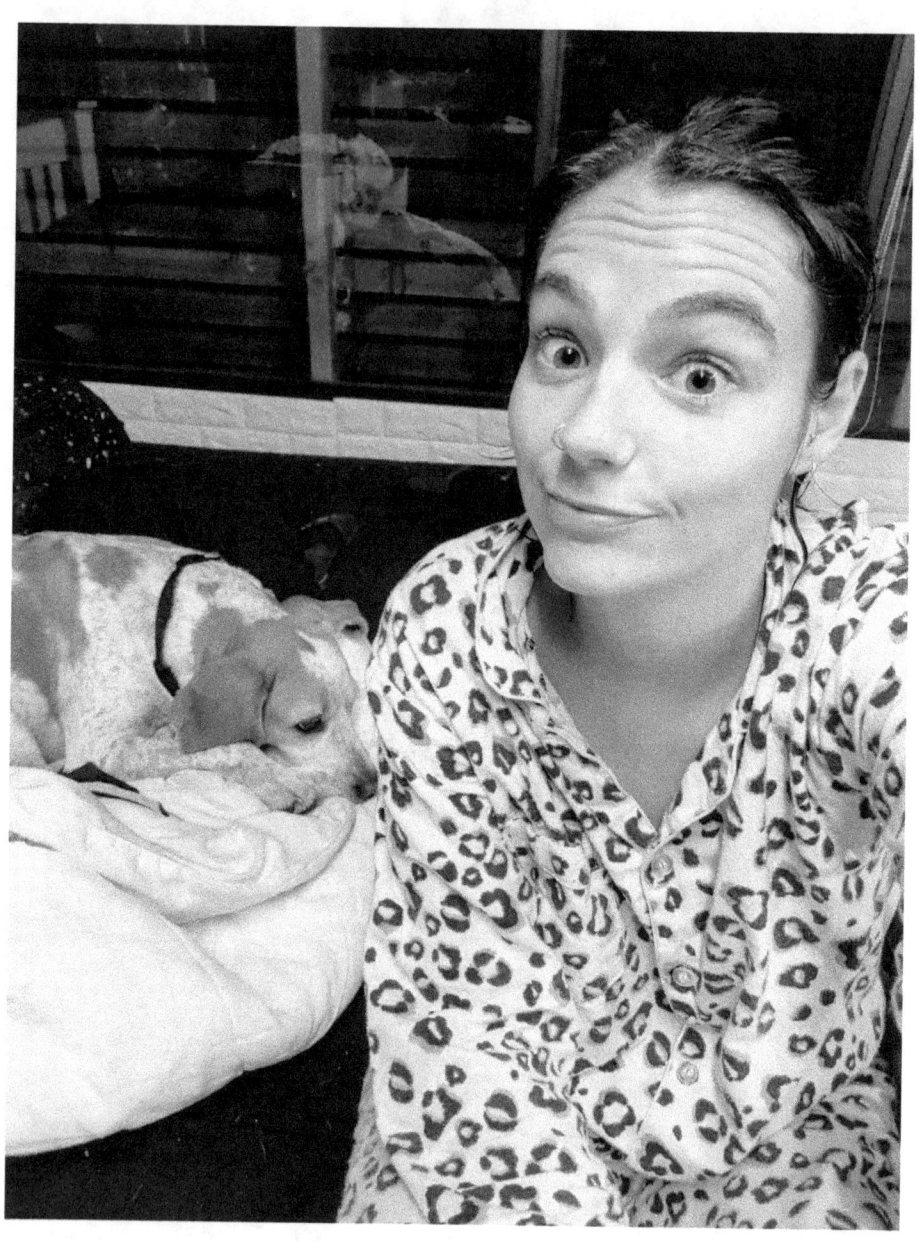

Dear Diary,

When I feel down, I do what I do best, I make a mess. Art for me is life; it's a window into my soul. I am a very expressive person; it is like a compulsion. I am not settled until what is inside is out, on paper, in paint or the words I speak. I cannot think of anything else until I do express the thoughts and feelings that consume me.

For a long time, I lost all that. I became so fearful of what people thought of me and my art I was too terrified even to start. I had to let go of that expectation and remind myself it didn't matter what others thought, that art meant something more to me than a picture to put on your wall. It is not a mere decoration. It is as an encryption to decode. A puzzle hiding and expressing my inner world. The tangled web of emotions that define me.

Art is just as important as the words I write or speak; it is my diary. It captures a moment in my life. A feeling or a thought. Without it, I am lost. Art fills the void where no words can tread. I often paint to put my feelings outside of my body and only then as they manifest on the canvas can I understand what they are. Their meaning often comes shortly after. I see the world in a range of colours, my thoughts are in pictures. I can remember things as clear as day replaying that moment like a video in my head. A photo seared into my mind; no detail too small to be forgotten. I see it all. Some of them still torment me. Others are there to unlock when I need a bit of sunshine. I envision my feelings in metaphors and analogies because that's how I see them in my mind. Like little scenes playing out in my head, like a mini movie with all the details you need to understand the setting and characters.

But sometimes these pieces of life become tangled up inside of me, until they create an entire world where nothing makes sense anymore. In these moments, I start feeling like time is running backwards – or maybe even forwards – while reality becomes more dreamlike by the second. It's this bizarre place where logic seems to exist and not exist, simultaneously throwing your brain into such confusion that it starts mixing up words too.

Perhaps that is why I have come to like abstract art. As a traditional artist I'd never really valued that style. It seemed to lack any form of talent with the absence of precision. Now I understand the need to let go of form and figures, to tap into pure expression. It is an emotion that cannot be defined, that needs to come out. It is not a portrait for anyone else but me. I do not try to make it aesthetically pleasing, although I think as a trained artist that comes naturally to me.

I just tap into the part of me that craves release. I am just the vessel of a force that needs to be painted. Each squiggly line and splash of colour tells a story of a part of my soul no one could possibly comprehend. Not even me.

Artist Barbie

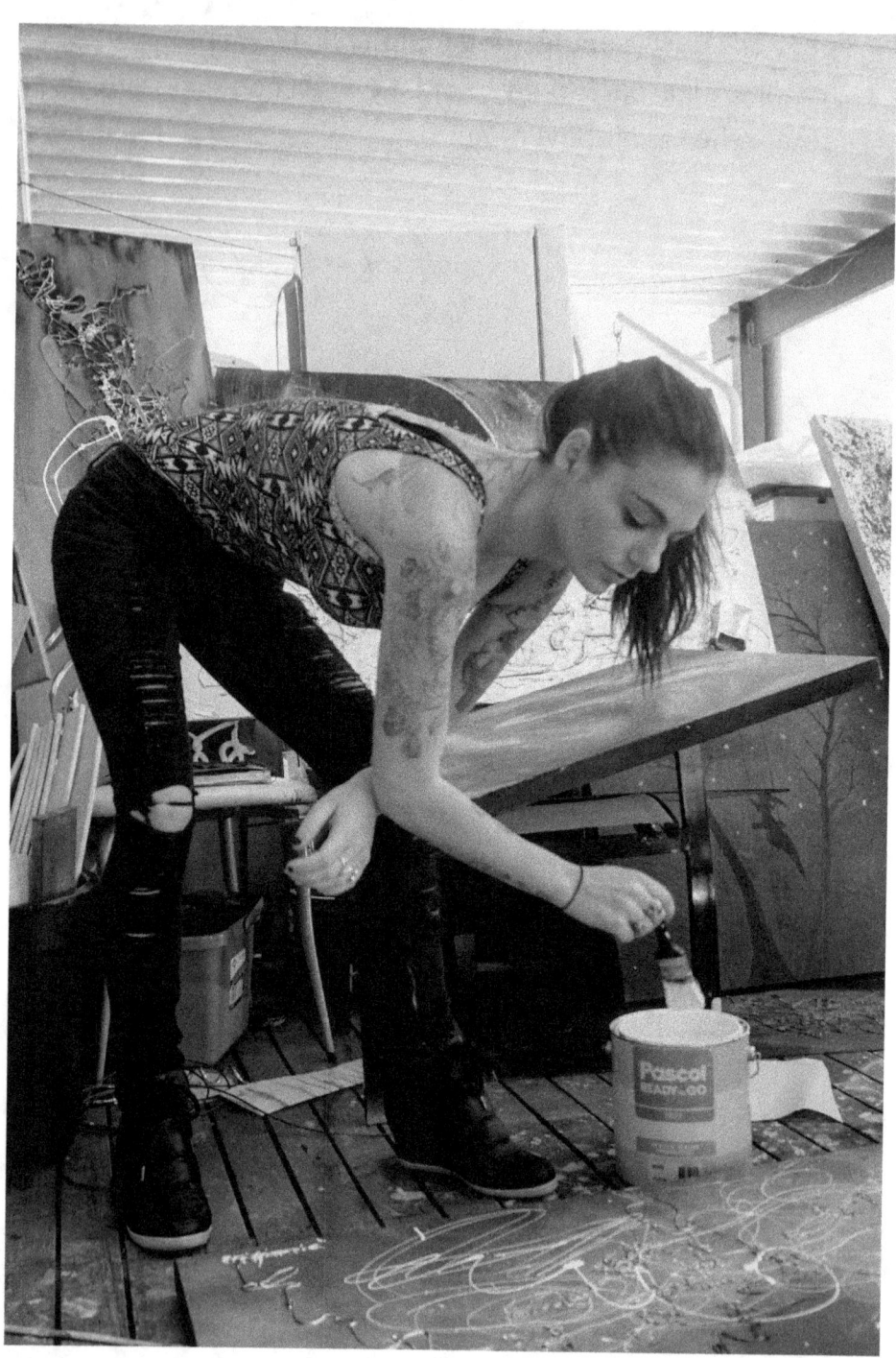

Dear Diary,

Remember when we were young and filled with joy, daydreaming about our future? When we honestly believed we could be whatever we wanted and nothing could stand in our way? The only obstacles we had were the ones right in front of us and like a champion horse, we could jump over anything that got in our way? Once upon a time I had faith in myself and faith that life would be kind to me. How wrong I was.

I realised tonight that my dreams don't fill me with joy anymore. Whenever I'm caught thinking of everything I ever wanted to be and still do, I am overwhelmed with incredible regret, anger, frustration and disappointment. I cannot see a future where life is kind. The only future I see is living like this for the rest of my life.

As I get older I realise there's a lot more standing in my way to becoming a ballerina, rock star, princess or any other childish hopes I may have had. Sure, there's an element of talent involved — hence no music career for me — but it's obvious that years of hard work and dedication are necessary to achieve some milestones. Success takes time and in an instantly gratified society where anything you want is at a touch of a button it's hard to see the point in trying at all.

As I age and watch the people around me

prosper in their chosen fields, I start to realise just how far behind I am. Starting ballet in your twenties seems preposterous!? Even allowing myself to want to become anything is incredibly naïve. The magnitude of the task ahead stops me from taking those first steps. I am chained to this heavy immoveable resistance that I can't seem to shake.

Who am I? Who do I want to be? Those are the thoughts that haunt me every single waking hour of the day.

Dreams children have and the faith that they have in them one day coming true is so sweet and innocent. It's a shame as they get older, reality hits and their goals get smaller. Suddenly the faith is lost. Hard work never really seems to pay off as promised and at first you think it's just a mistake, a giant misunderstanding, a glitch in the matrix. You begin to question the universe's grand plan. You spend what feels like a lifetime trying to correct yourself based on the premise that you are broken or simply not enough. The life you seek seems so far out of reach. Fairy tales aren't real, life isn't a movie plot and we don't always get what we want. But that was all easier to swallow when I dreamt of fantasies so grand even Harry Potter wouldn't believe them possible.

As I grow older, I am encouraged to start managing my expectations. I was told to pull my head out from the clouds and stop stargazing. I was ordered to strive towards things that others thought possible. I am not sure if this is just from the opinion of someone riddled with mental illness or if we all feel this way. There was a time in my life when I believed there was a chance all of my wildest dreams could come true. Back in a time when I hadn't tried to achieve them and failure wasn't in my vocabulary. Even when I first tasted the bitterness of failure I still had the sweet taste of success lingering on my tongue. Until mental illness struck. Pretty soon my failures outweighed my success stories. Until I felt like I'd never succeed at anything ever again.

"You could achieve anything you want if you just tried," they told me. As if they had identified the problem and found an easy solution. I *had* been trying. But no matter how hard I try; success always falls through my fingers. The cracks begin to show. Each time I failed the more faith I lost in myself. Until even dreaming about a more appealing future made me depressed. The thoughts of things I'd never have followed me around like a bad smell.

"Lower your goals and aspirations," they all suggested. What is the point in living a life you do not want? Why design a mediocre existence? Was I not born to stand out? How could they expect me to accept being like this for the rest of my life?

Nonetheless, I did what they all told me to do,

I lowered my expectations. So low in fact, it's pathetically sad. The things I yearn for are so simple yet unattainable. Things like having a symptom-free day, managing to tidy my room, take a shower, wash some dishes and get out of bed. I just want a day where I feel happy and can be free from the torment of expectation, my past traumas and the self-loathing voice in my mind. That's all I ask. Just for a day.

The fact that I have failed to achieve even those simple things is so depressing. After years of trying, years of fighting, years of yearning to just have a clean slate. Any plans I make past this moment right now only set me up for more disappointment. Any person I count on leaves me feeling heartbroken and betrayed. Even myself. They say you are your own worst enemy and with me that must be the case.

I don't think it's tooting your own horn to know what you're capable of being. The things I want – even my wildest dreams – I know I could actually achieve. That is, if I wasn't mentally ill. The sick version of me will achieve nothing. She will destroy more than she can help build. Her highest aspirations are to take her medication on time, make sure she has enough scripts and doesn't run out, and function in a way that remotely resembles a living person instead of a drowned raccoon shivering to death.

I guess the question I grapple with is, if I've

been that person for so many years, how do I know it's just my illness and not who I am? I've spent my whole life since everything fell apart trying to get back to the person I was. But I don't think you can ever go back.

I'm not sure what was worse ... realising I am most likely never going to achieve any of my dreams, or the fact that the biggest obstacle that stands in my way is myself. Tears well in my eyes each time I am faced with the terrifying truth that I may never be happy because of who I am. When I'm in a really bad episode I cope by daring not to dream. It's deadly. Because nothing sends me towards suicide faster than feeling like there's no point to life. If I will never achieve anything I set out to do, what's the point in living at all?

The older I get, the louder the clock inside my head begins to tick. They say your youth is the best time of your life. Well what if it's the worst?

"One day you'll get to where you want to be, one day you will be happy and be able to start living again" they keep assuring me. Although there is nothing reassuring about it. What if I sort myself by the time I'm 30 or 40? Isn't your life over then anyway? You're past your professional and physical prime. So what's the point of even beginning to work hard now if it's just to maybe one day, someday actually enjoy myself for the first time? This isn't living. This isn't life. This has to be some sort of illusion of my mind.

P.S: Don't worry about me, I'm fine. Just a snippet from my daily inner dialogue.

Expectation Barbie

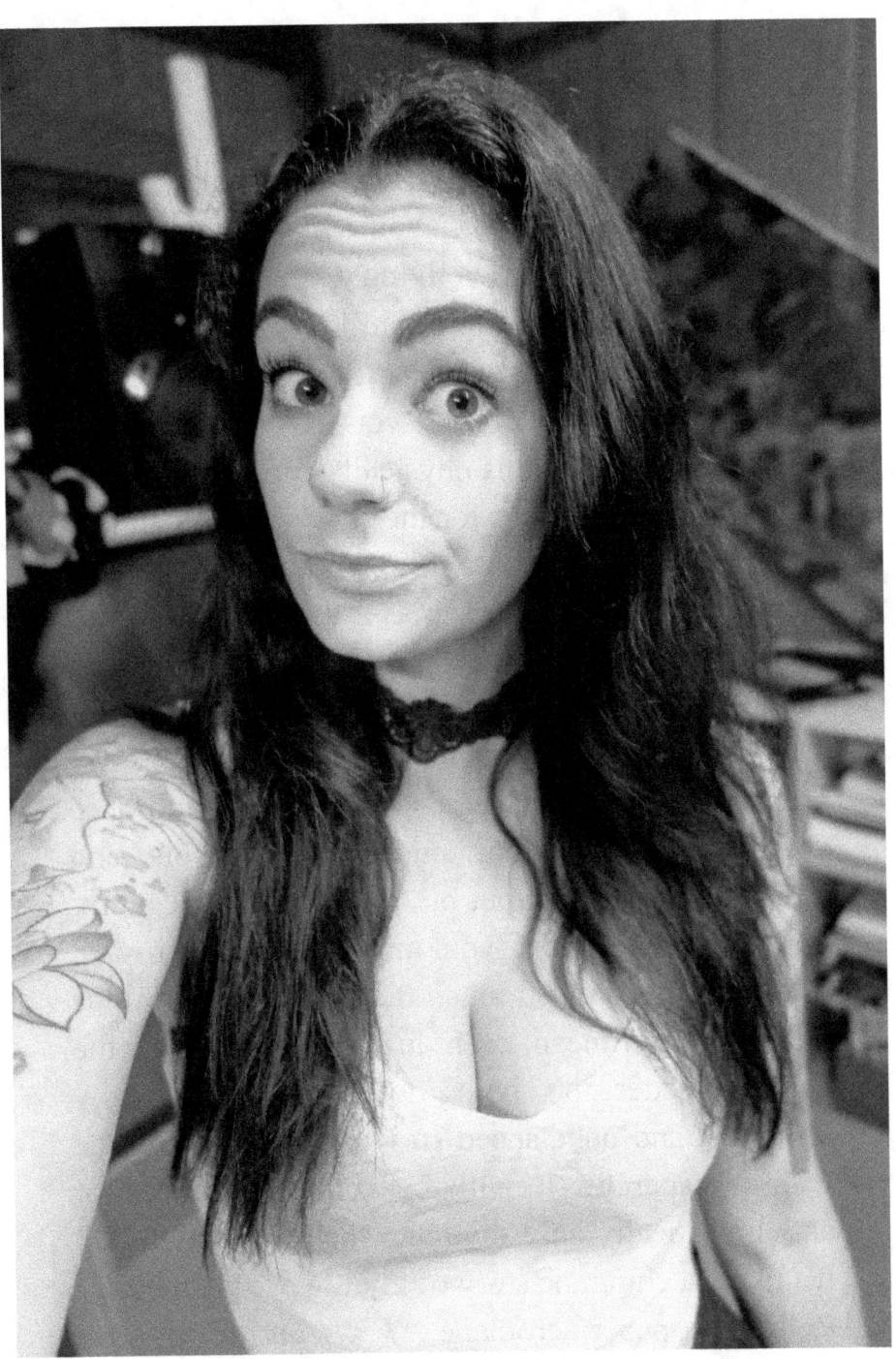

Dear Diary,

It pisses me off immensely when they say, "mental illness is treatable", like it's a common cold that'll pass in a few days or a scratch that will heal on its own without a scar. "You will get better!" they preach, like it's as easy as flying a kite.

Although operating a kite is hard as shit! Has anyone ever done it well? I mean there's a lot that goes into it. First of all, you have to have an aerodynamic kite that is physically capable of flying. Which is only possible for the first time you slide it out of the plastic placenta it was birthed in at the kite factory. Usually Christmas day. But you're immediately fucked once it's kinked and crinkled, usually after it's been trodden on and cast aside for years or someone hasn't packed it into the car properly. It probably has a few holes in it too once you fish it out from under the scrabble and monopoly boxes you put on top of it. So if it's torn, then it's broken, and you might as well throw it away. There's only so much duct tape can do in this world. Cause I mean, even duct tape won't make the kite fly better; it's going to be aerodynamically imperfect and unbalanced so like a paper aeroplane with a paperclip it will fly round in circles or anticlimactically nose dive into the ground. SPLAT! It's like watching the story of my life every time I try to throw a paper aeroplane. *YES! Houston we have to lift off! NAWWWWW looks like another Apollo disaster, might as well throw the aircraft away.* Unfortunately, the only difference between my mind and a kite is that I can't throw that away ... blow it away perhaps ... (insert thinking emoji) but then my kite will never fly ...

So let's say you have a brand new perfectly in order kite. The conditions have to be perfect to fly it too. If there's no wind, well you're up shit creek without a paddle. Too much wind and you're in the middle of the ocean in a tropical cyclone holding on to a whale-sized helium balloon about to be sucked up into the vortex. Or you're just that idiot at the beach being dragged through the sandstorm trying to tame your kite. Maybe you think you look like Hercules wrangling the three-headed hydra to victory. At least until you remember you're just an idiot on the beach trying to fly a kite and failing miserably.

I think it's better to leave the kite flying to the expert kite enthusiasts that rock up and put your crappy dollar store rainbow kite to shame with their flaming dragon jumbo jet kites dancing in the sky with ease. You know, the ones that have a harness wrapped around their waist and at least two handles attached to the kite so that they can direct it with accuracy in the sky?

Watch how quickly a beach clears with fathers

retreating into their SUVs once they get wind of those guys! Nothing deflates a man's ego quicker than not being able to get it up. Kites, I mean. I only just realised how closely kites resemble me. Not because men can't get it up, but because although mental illness recovery *may* be possible, it's *not* easy! To begin with, my kite is already broken, and I only have one! I can't just walk into a thrift shop and buy a new brain for $1. Maybe one day when we are all androids that might be possible, but for now we are restricted by the limitations of our human form.

After all this time actively seeking treatment I know all too well that it *is* as simple as flying a kite. Because operating a kite is *not* simple and sometimes you wish you could take it out in a thunderstorm hoping for that bolt of lightning to strike for a quick and shocking end! Or perhaps it will just work just as well as the clinical procedure Electroconvulsive Therapy. Perhaps lightning will have the same effect as ETC, passing not so carefully controlled electric currents through the brain to relieve depression and psychosis? I would have more chance of being cured by lightning than the severely inadequate mental healthcare system. Maybe then I wouldn't be punished/stigmatised/frowned upon/judged so harshly for simply not being okay.

I know it's hard to believe. I never wanted to

believe it. I guess others wouldn't either until they experienced it. Or just shut the fuck up for two seconds and took the time to listen to someone talk about it. Perhaps with an open mind …

But I know I'm asking too much. It just seems everyone has something to say, but nobody wants to listen. I must admit I'm often the same. I'm not an insensitive, ignorant asshole, but when people talk, I am usually already planning my reply before they even stop talking.

Note to self: Start listening more.

Note to self: Find interesting people to listen to.

Kite Flying Barbie

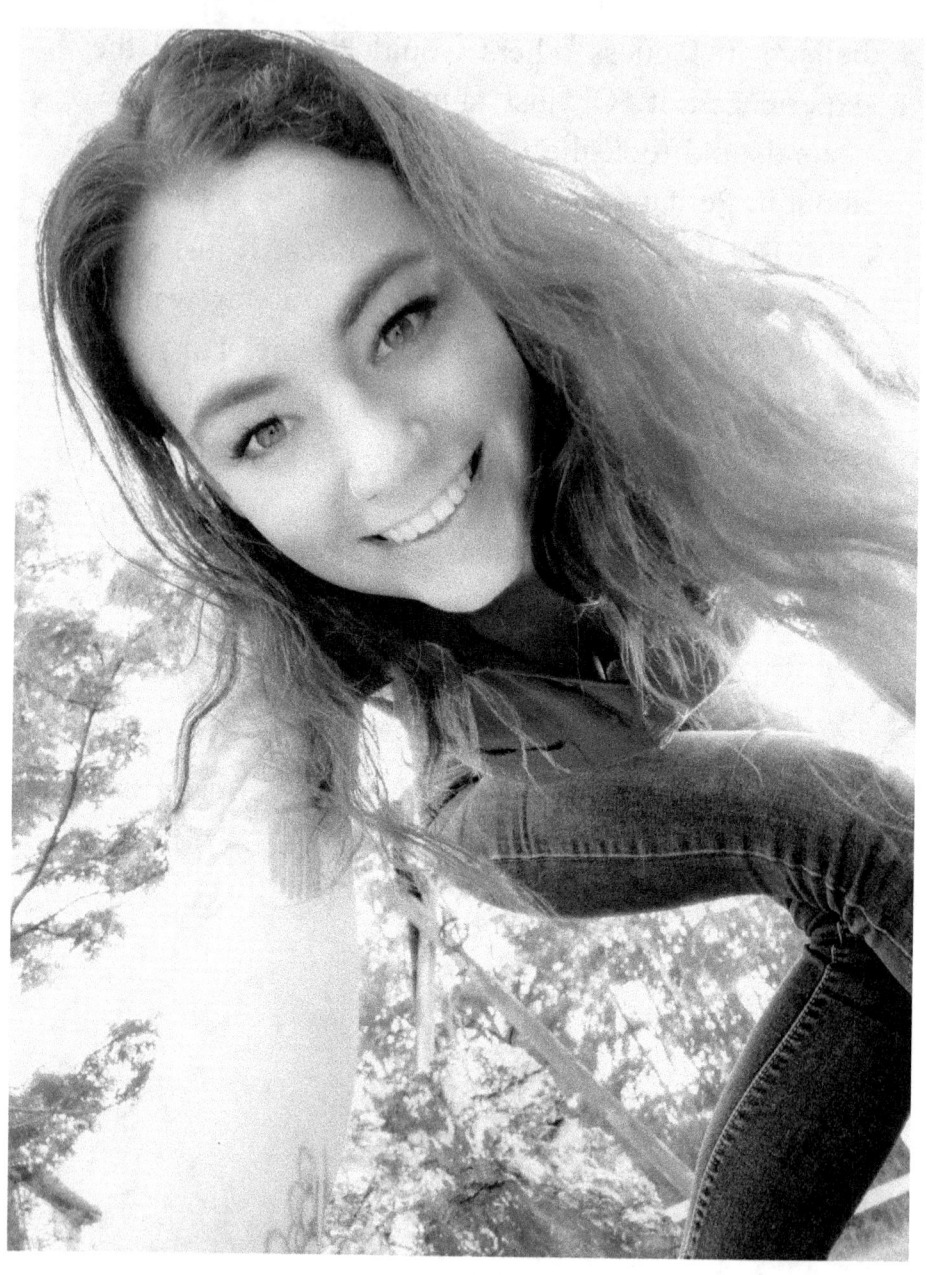

Dear Diary,

I cried all the way home today. I let it all out on the canvas, and I felt good. Then I stubbed my toe, drank a fly that drowned in my coffee and got eaten alive by mosquitos under my house as I painted. I cried again, felt crappy and then cleaned my room for a few hours. Not sure why it took so long. Do I really make that much mess? Or do I just get distracted and do pointless things that make me feel productive but don't actually get me anywhere? I felt crappy again, so I laid in bed for a while until I found the motivation to take Northy for a walk on the beach. The sun was shining bright, and I danced on the beach alone because nobody is ever at the beaches here. I love it. It made me feel good again.

I don't remember exactly why, but by the time I got home I felt so shit again. I had a massive migraine and climbed into bed, completely pissed off by the heat wave that had hit late afternoon. The smell of rain was in the air, but that just made it sticky and muggy. My housemate was burning incense, and normally I love the hippy smell of this place, but it wasn't helping my migraine. I'd switched between crappy, to good and then everything in between all day. One minute I was cleaning my room and doing all my washing. Sorting my stuff out *like a boss* and the next I was like "URGHHHH! I fucking hate my life!" Then I was back on a high, buying three canvases and painting again. *Yay!* Then I wanted to cut myself again. Then suddenly I was listening to music, cleaning, and dancing around in my underwear in the rain like a lunatic. Then again I was back to "ugh life!" Then painting again. Then I had dinner and took myself out after with Northy for a drive. I ended up at the local jetty and had such a pleasant time down by the water with my baby boy. The fresh air and the cool ocean breeze was calming and soothing to me.

Artist Barbie

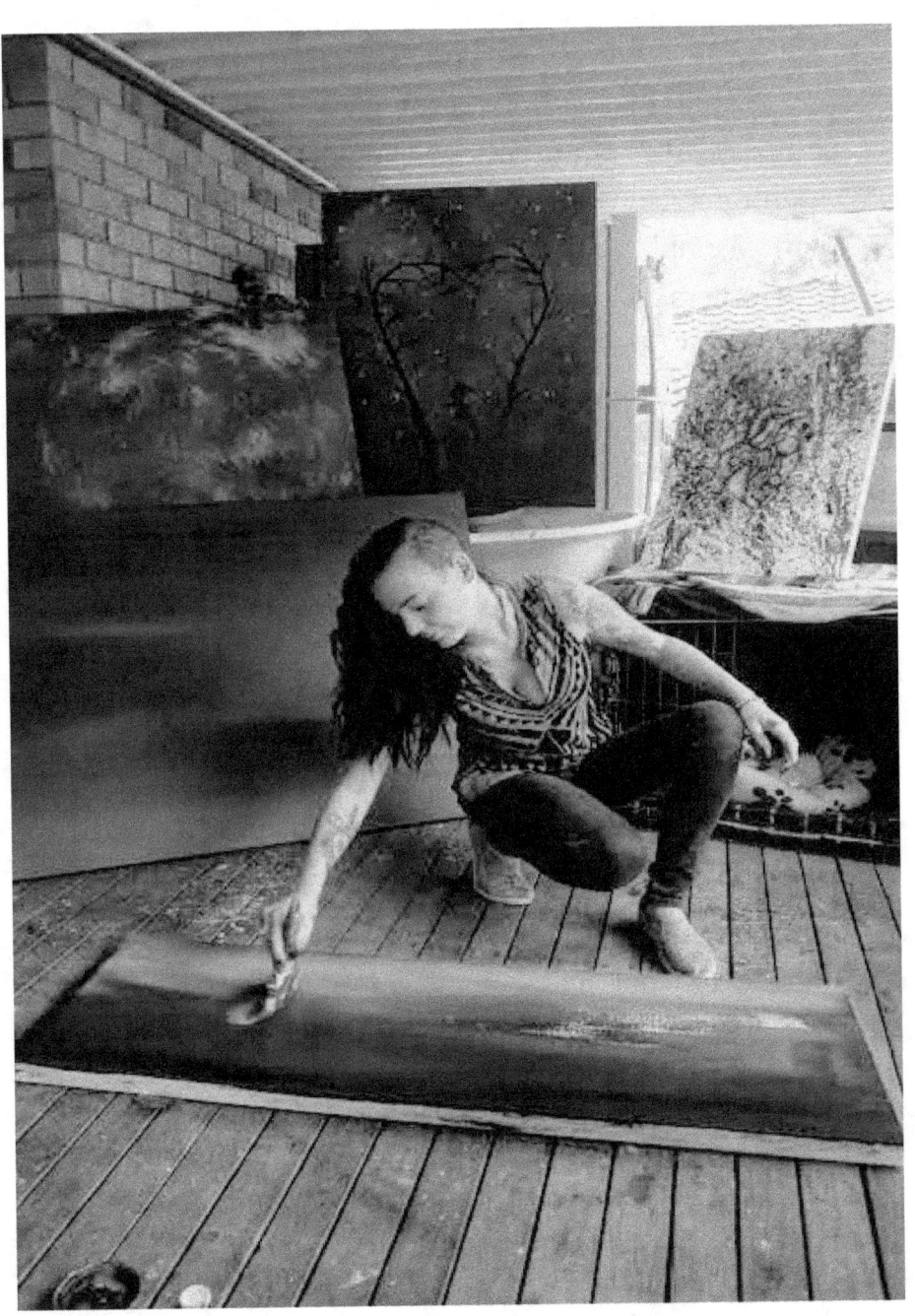

Dear Diary,

I think half of the reason I struggle is because I compare my 'behind the scenes' with everyone else's 'highlight reel'. I don't think it's just social media's fault. We only pick the highlights of our life to share with others, partly because there just isn't enough time to say it all but also because we would rather hide the feeling of hopelessness rather than reaching out and being burnt.

We are all comparing ourselves to each other because we think life is this giant competition and there is only one way to win. What is it that we win anyway? Is it really recognition? Or does that represent something else? All I want is to be loved. But I think that is both an internal and an external battle. It's a chicken and the egg scenario. What is it with chickens anyway? Why do people care so much about them? We are obsessed with what came first or why the chicken crossed the road, but no other animals are put under such scrutiny. I dream of a world where chickens can cross the road without having their motives questioned.

I wish I could go through a day without questioning myself too. I spend almost every second of every day in this internal tug of war with myself. It's an ongoing debate of whether or not I am worthy. I hated who I was and struggled so much with insecurities. I still do because everyone I ever cared about convinced me I was wrong, a monster, an outcast, a disgusting excuse for a human being. They planted the seeds inside me to fester like a cancerous disease that infiltrated every cell in my body. It reminds me of this science experiment we learnt about at school where parents tried to point out that heavy metal music was damaging to young minds. They did tests on plants concluding that if you say nice things to them, they will flourish and grow. If you talk to them with hate, they will wither and die. That's what happened to me on the inside. Underneath my shiny facade, I am just a withered brown dying mung bean plant. I wonder if it is the doubt that killed them too? Or did they simply lose the will to live because they weren't appreciated? I think cells just lose the essence of life when they don't see a point in living it. Who would want to grow in an environment that doesn't appreciate them? What are you even growing for? There isn't a light at the end of the tunnel because either way you are going to be fucked up.

    I have to fix myself from the inside out to rid myself of doubt. I know this is something that will take considerable time. I have to undo years of programming to embrace my uniqueness and love my differences. Time is something I have. But I must be cautious with this time. I don't want to feed the cancer as I try to fight it back. I have identified how it grows, what gives it oxygen and food. So That's why for now I shut myself off to the world emotionally to starve it. I physically go about my business, but I put up a wall. Not to push others away although I know that is a consequence. But to make sure I don't feed this cancerous form inside my aching soul. I must be stronger than the life force threatening to tear me apart. I'm alive on the outside. I'm almost dead on the inside. This is my last chance to save my life. To finally have a life. I must feel alive and want to live. That is my mission. To make me whole again.

    I am selfish for once In my life by necessity. I must do things for me. Because I've spent too long doing them for everyone else, I neglected to attend to the damage being done within. Life is too short and precious to be eternally unhappy.

Self-Isolating Barbie

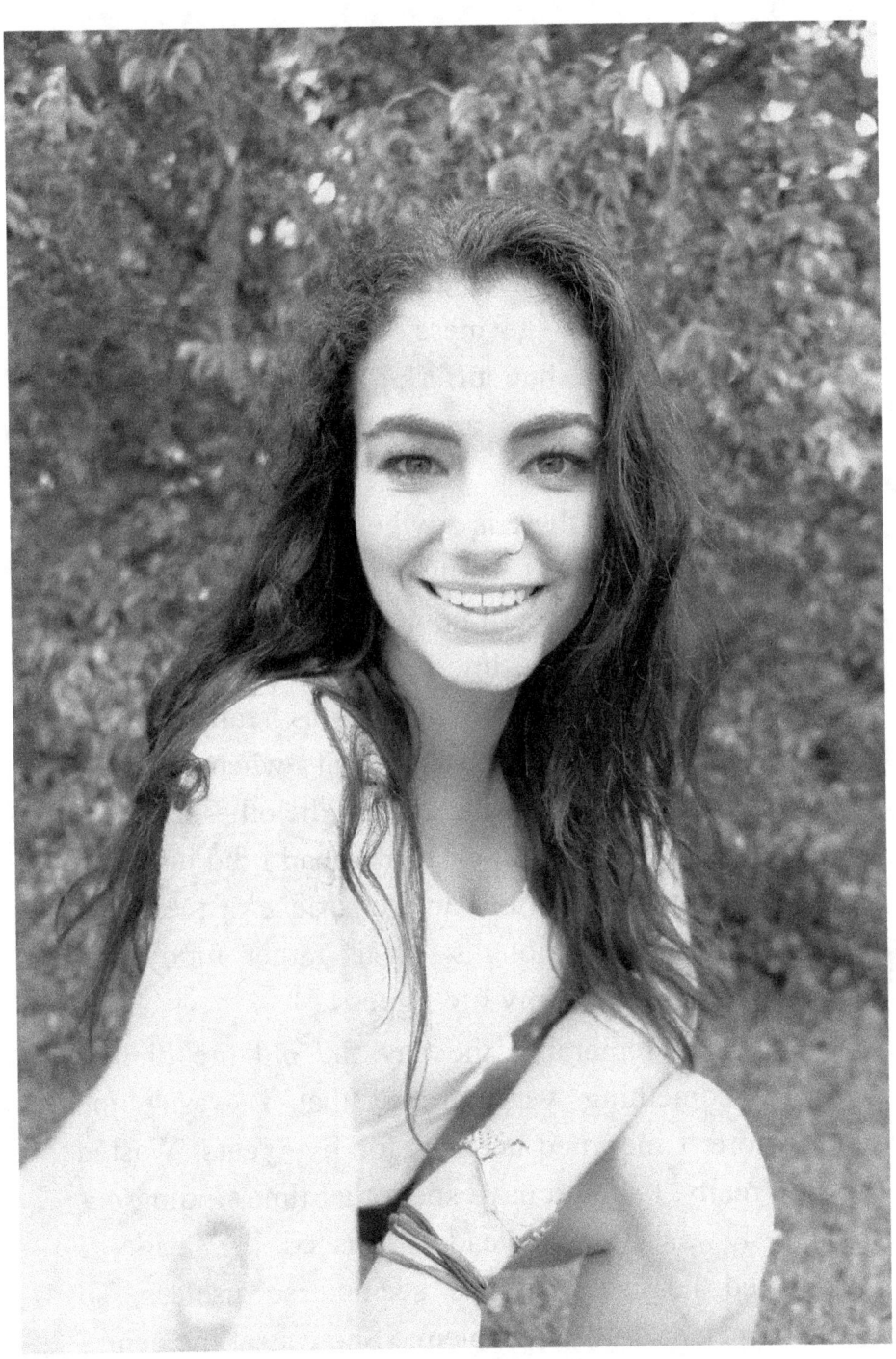

Dear Diary,

I am always incredibly affected by things outside of my control. I was always very proactive in changing the things I could change, so I ponder how to escape or handle the things people throw at me: I could sob on my knees and worry about how I'm going to clean up the mess, or remind myself that pain is inevitable, but suffering is optional. That our failures and struggles are there to teach valuable lessons.

Sometimes there is nowhere to run, nowhere to hide. While we can't always control the things that trouble us, we can learn how to cope with distress. I often think back to a time I remember being happy. Childhood for a time. When I was really little, I sometimes used to make leaf boats when it rained and floated them down the gutter. The other day on a wonderful bush walk to clear my head I did just that. I watched the boats float on the surface of the water before it sank. I thought it was rather funny and poetic. The story of my life I guess.

I can remember the day the old me died. I knew something was wrong, that I wasn't me anymore. I mourned her loss for five years. Wasted time really. I should have spent that time finding out who I was now. Instead, I pushed her aside, I rejected her because she seemed so useless, so incompetent. Full of problems. She was at the centre of them all. Everything seemed to be going wrong and just when I thought it had been the worst year of my life. The next was even worse. "Next year will be better," everyone preached. I always had hope. But I know better now.

Pain is expected, mental breakdowns are inevitable and sometimes completely out of my control. I've had to change the way I live my life to accommodate this new person. I thought she was ugly, hideous and unlovable. A monster under the skin. I watched everyone shy away from me as I slunk back into the shadows. I wasn't even mad, I envied them. I wish I had the choice to run away from myself. I did try for a time; I had wanted to get my old self back. She was awesome. She kicked ass. She succeeded at whatever she set her mind to. Losing her was a horrific loss, like grieving a loved one.

I now realise I was me all along. I'd just lost the version of me everyone else loved. The me I cherished as a child was crippled with overwhelming failure and inadequacy. The people in my life didn't help. "What's wrong with you?" they asked. "This isn't you, go back to being yourself." They didn't realise I couldn't. They didn't know how hard I tried. How many times I cried. Failure wasn't me, yet it followed me wherever I went.

It was only last year I spent some time getting

to know the new me. Funnily enough, she wasn't all that bad. Sure, it took me some time to realise that, especially when I was surrounded by people who didn't appreciate what I had to offer. I realised I was more like my childhood self with the same ambitions I'd had as a very young child. I wanted to give speeches, I wanted to write a book, I wanted to be an artist, and I wanted to change the world. I realised that even my illness wasn't all that bad. In actual fact, it had given me everything I wanted as a child. Sure I had lost what I wanted after school, but maybe that wasn't what I'd really wanted at all. Can you believe I actually gave up writing at about fourteen?

So how am I going about learning to love who I am? Well, right now I'd settle for even liking who I am! First of all, I had to identify and eliminate all the people in my life that made me feel shit about myself. It doesn't matter how much you love someone, if they are unhealthy for you they have to go. Then I reminded myself every day what makes me a valuable person. I start by getting the people I trust in my life to tell me all the things they value and appreciate about me! That helps give me some inspiration to remember those things if ever in doubt! I also have to practice acceptance. I have to accept I am mentally ill and everything that has happened in my life as a result. This is incredibly hard. But I look back on my life and see five lost years. I am not going to lose another five! I have to get on top of my shit. I just have to. Regardless of how I got here, I am in this mess, and no one else is going to clean it up. I have to push through and deal with it, even if I have to do it on my own. I've sought help from doctors and therapists and have done a lot of self-reflection and soul searching. I take ownership of my life (even the things people have done to me) because yes it is my fault: I let them. I had the power to throw them out of my life, but I didn't. I wish I knew I had the power to do that at the time. But I am stronger now, I know better. Then after a time of isolation, I have opened myself up to the world again. I find this very hard. It is incredible the power positive and healthy people can have on your life.

Affirmation of my self-worth is relatively meaningless from friends and the like. My self-worth is heavily attached to a partner's approval of me. Normally I fall for narcissistic, unhealthy manipulators. I guess I feel it's a challenge to win their affection. I didn't think I had it in me to spot them on approach before they got their hooks into me and I couldn't let go. But maybe I have that awareness now. I realised in shutting everyone out, I also shut out the possibility of someone being good for me. Someone who is encouraging, accommodating, understanding and incredibly validating. At first I thought, *how can anyone be good for me? People are evil, they all cause pain.* But now I know that's not true. We just have to be aware of the warning signs and maintain our boundaries and proceed with our eyes wide open. Do it carefully, but do it when the time is right, or when you find someone that is just right. Someone who encourages you to be whoever you want to be and appreciates you for who you are and praises you for the wonderful person you are. Someone who likes the real you so much you start to like yourself too!

Barbie

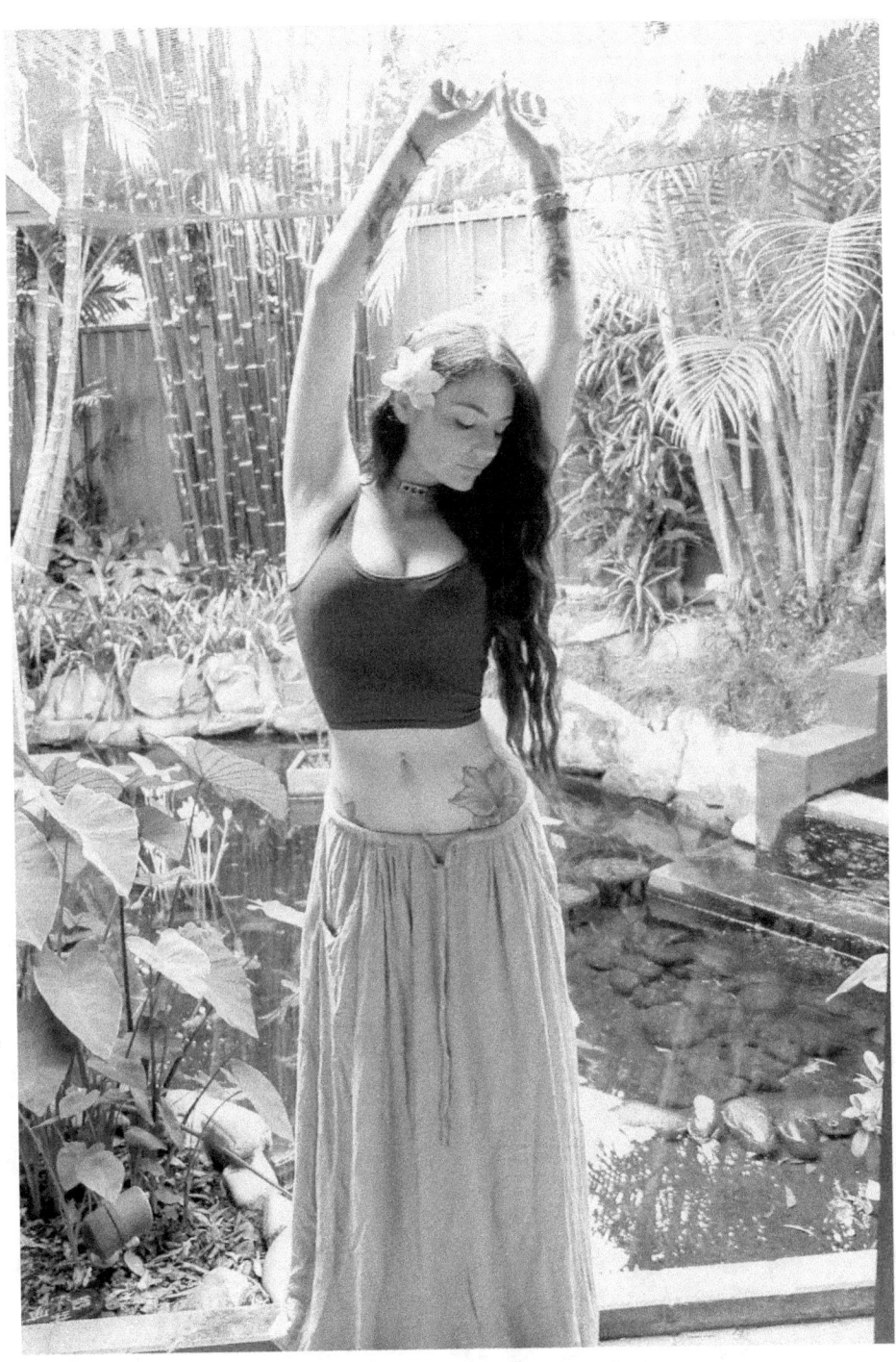

I needed a hero so a Hero I became

Bipolar Barbie

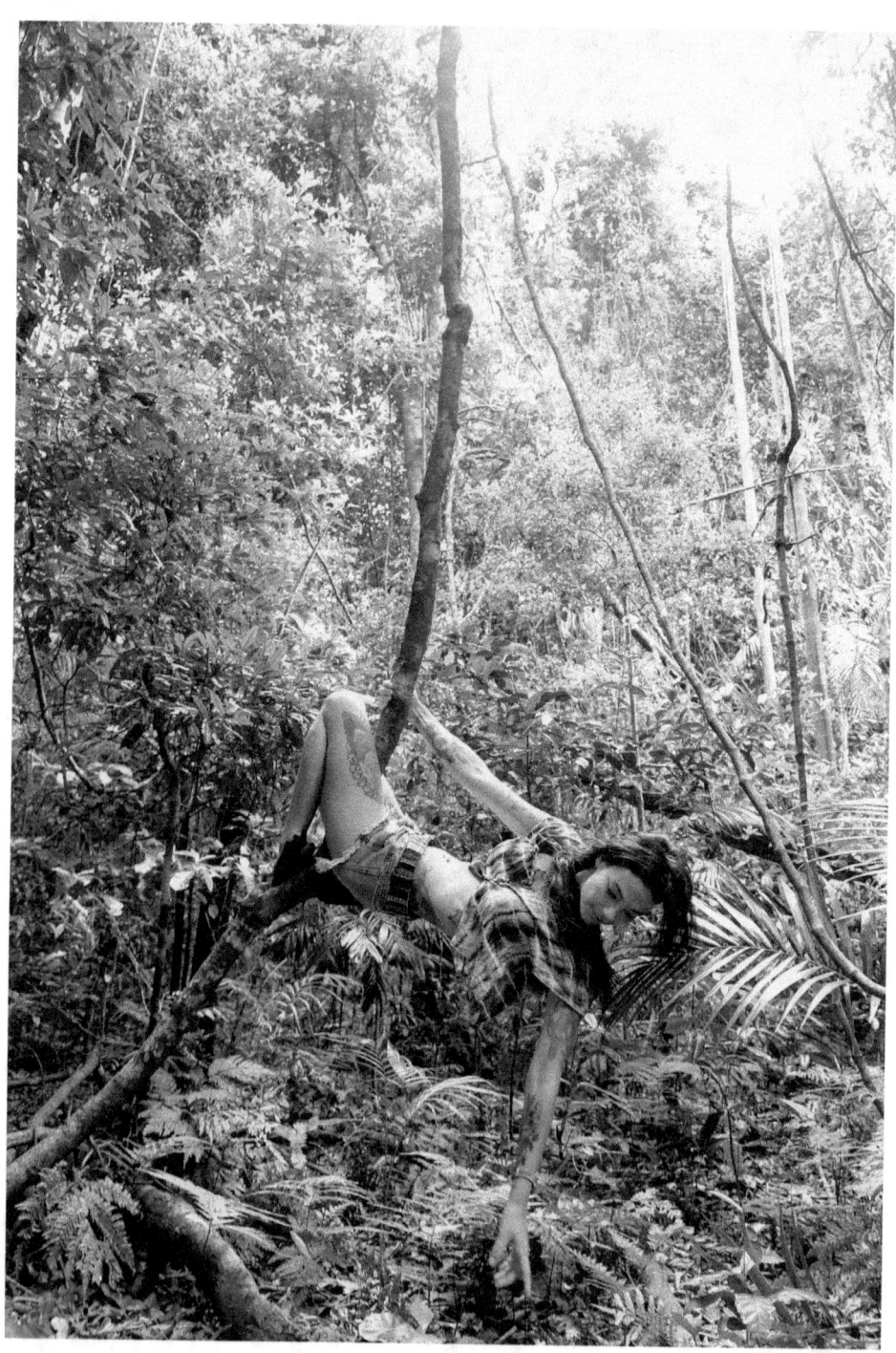

Dear Diary,

When I first became mentally ill, I had no idea what was going on. It was like I was sucked up in this tornado then dumped down a rabbit hole. I had no idea where I was. It was like I lost myself overnight. Every part of me that I adored was gone. I was stripped of all that I was and I had no idea who I had become. All I knew was that I couldn't function. All I could think was that there had to be a reason for this pai.? A method to this madness. I thought, *If there is a God, he has to have a plan that makes all of this worth it in the end. Otherwise, this is just a sick joke the almighty creator enjoys torturing me with.*

I tried to figure out what was going on because I knew something was very wrong. But I don't think anyone had ever explained mental illness to me in a way that would help me identify whether I was suffering from one. I felt so helpless. I was just wandering around saying, "Guys, I'm not okay", but I couldn't really tell people I wasn't okay because I didn't know why I wasn't.

I couldn't quite put my finger on it. Something just didn't feel right. It was like I was trapped in a cage. I couldn't escape. I was bound with my hands behind my back. I couldn't do anything I used to be able to do. I was being held back by this beast no one else could see. They just kept telling me to get on with my life. To suck it up and deal with it. They were angry and frustrated with me. They didn't understand why I couldn't just go back to the life I had before. They demanded results but refused to ask the right questions. I didn't have answers to them anyway, I was scratching my head trying to figure out what was going on. But it would have been nice if I didn't have to figure it out alone.

My journey would have been a hell of a lot easier if people had known how to help me or even showed an interest in doing so. The road is tough enough, I really resent having to go it alone. I didn't know who to turn to and when I reached out to people they didn't really know what to do either.

I don't think you really can comprehend how valuable your sanity is until you've lost it. You don't realise how much of a huge part of your existence your sanity is. I think without it you can't function; you can't even hope to function in our society.

I knew that something was wrong, but I didn't want to admit it. That's why it really annoys me when people accuse me of just deciding to have a mental illness. As if I want to be mentally ill? But in the same conversation those same people deny that I am sick. To think I had just chosen to suddenly destroy my life is a mind blowing accusation I have never understood.

Symptoms of my illness and how they manifest

in my life are just pushed aside as poor life choices. I was convinced by everybody that how I was feeling was normal. No one seemed to grasp the gravity of the situation.

For the record, being suicidal is really not normal!

It's scary and incredibly brave to put your hand up and admit that you need help, but it's even more terrifying to not get any. We can raise awareness through slogans to reach out, but what if there is no one to reach out to?

No one told me to see a doctor or a therapist. No one knew what to do with me besides assuring me I would be alright and it would pass or encouraging me to just suck it up and deal with it. I had been feeling this way for a really long time, so to then be told just to ride it out when that's all I had been doing for months made no sense to me at all.

A lot of people use the excuse that they didn't know how to help. But the only way you know how is to talk to me. It's a conversation not many want to have. But it's an important one that can save lives. I know it can be scary, but not knowing how to do something isn't an excuse. There is plenty of information out there on the internet. It's pretty easy to *Google* anything these days.

I believe in starting conversations about mental

health because I think any conversation can be a life-changing one. I bring it up in everyday conversation and it blows my mind how many people start talking about their mental health simply because I've brought it up. I don't do it in a really obvious way. I don't force it on anyone, I just casually mention it in passing conversations. I don't even mean to do it. I'm not ashamed.

When people ask me why I talk about my mental health so openly, I just think, *It never occurred to me not to!* I think it is something we should talk about and I think most people really want to talk about it. They are just scared to start. All it takes is for one person to take the initiative and suddenly a door opens up, an opportunity to talk about something that could save the life of someone you care about. A conversation I wish I could have with some friends but will never be able to have because it's too late.

Most people are afraid of being judged, but I was being judged long before I started talking about my mental health. Maybe people feel they can open up to me particularly because they know I won't be judgmental. I will accept them and their illness if that's a part of them. I won't invalidate them; I won't tell them that it's easy because I know for a fact that it's not. I won't sugar coat anything.

I have gone out of my way to find treatment,

and to find people that can actually help me so that I might be able to point those who need help in the right direction. But at the same time, I'm not going to tell them that my direction is the only direction. It really is a journey that you have to take on your own. It took me five years to really figure out what "it" was.

First I was diagnosed with Anxiety and Depression. Then Bipolar Disorder and Anxiety and then Bipolar Disorder, Anxiety and Borderline Personality Disorder, and then the additional diagnosis of Premenstrual Dysphoric Disorder. Who knows what my diagnosis might be next? Maybe this diagnosis is final, maybe it's not. I don't think anyone really knows what's going on. It's something I am going to have to re-evaluate time and time again. I'm constantly changing and my symptoms are too. They manifest in different areas of my life. The more I learn, the greater the understanding I have of the beast that lives within.

I believe in using everything and anything at my disposal to help me get my life back. I don't just rely on medication. I don't just rely on therapy; it's a lifestyle change as well. However I do believe that there is one universal truth that applies to anyone who is struggling. It was only when I stopped fighting my mental illness and started working with it, did I begin to find any relief. Only when I stopped rejecting it and trying to push it away, could I embrace it to heal.

I had to learn that I have a certain handicap. (Fuck everyone who wants to tell me I don't have one.) I'm not going to be able to function all year round. I can't work full-time no matter how hard I try to. I knew that there would be stormy seas ahead. I knew that there would be days where I felt helpless and I was held underwater. I knew that it wouldn't be smooth sailing. I knew that I would get lost and the currents would pull me back and forth and I would drift further away from shore than I wanted to be. As long as I could see that land; that was what I was working towards. I had never been so determined to get there; I had faith that one day I eventually would.

Finally, to my surprise, after scanning the well-known barren horizon I caught a glimpse of land! This was the crossroads I recently experienced. The strength in accepting that no one was going to save me; it didn't matter if they didn't want to, or just couldn't. Focusing on getting those answers didn't matter. I had to save myself. I had found a glimpse of land, and I knew that was where I wanted to be headed.

I made a choice, despite the long and exhausting journey ahead, to lift my arms out of the water and put my head down to swim. I now have my goal on the horizon, a direction I wish to head. This has given me faith; one day I will get there, as long as I can see land. But I am also well aware that the current will take me back at times or send me sideways so that I may feel like I'm swimming and getting nowhere. The struggles will still be there, and at times the wind will pick up, and the waves will begin to rage, and I will lose sight of land. But I now have faith that it exists.

I have seen what life could be like on the horizon and I am more determined than ever before to fight for my life. I can't wait for the moment I sit with my loyal companion on the shore and silently observe how far I've come. I feel empowered by the idea that when I finally do greet my friends and family on shore, I can tell them I did this on my own.

There is a lot I have learned since those days at law school. For the first time in my life, I have deliberately shut out nearly everything but myself, because I've realised there's a lot more that can hurt my mood than just biochemistry. Shitty relationships, life stresses and all the fucking baggage that goes along with mental illness. Not all of it has to be there. Even the things you feel need to be there the most probably don't. I was lucky, tragically it was all taken away from me. I was reluctant at the time, but now I see it's the best thing that ever happened to me.

If I needed a hero and no one was around then I was going to have to become my own hero.

Empowered Barbie

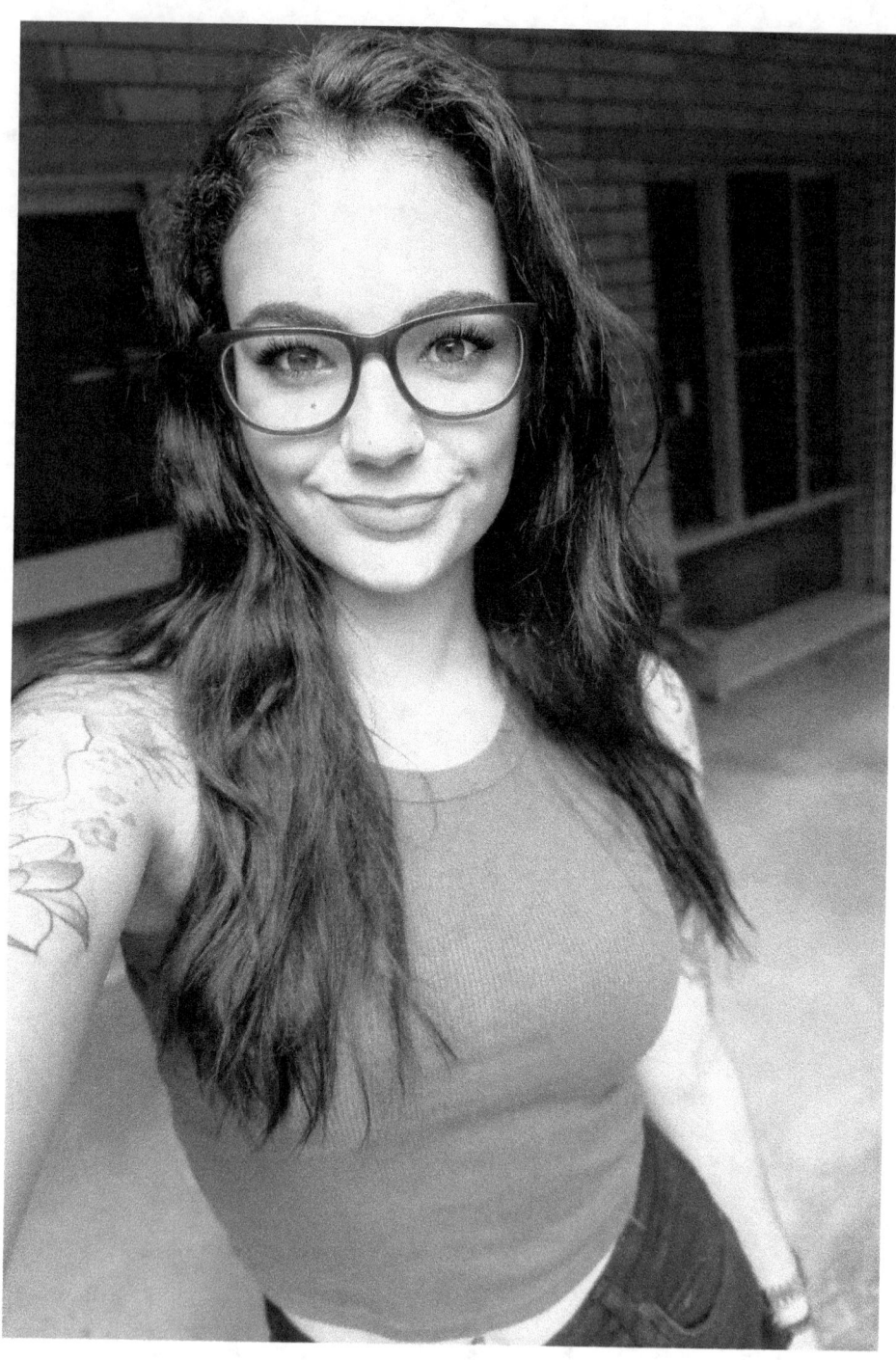

ABOUT THE AUTHOR

Bipolar Barbie is a young Australian Artist, Author and Motivational Speaker. When people ask her why she decided to talk about her mental health issues publicly she responds "It never occurred to me not to!"

She started out as a social media influencer on Instagram and YouTube becoming known worldwide for giving a "Creative take on living with Mental Illness". Expressing herself in a raw, honest and relatable way. She says her qualifications are "Lived Experience". She blogs about her journey to overcome with homelessness, bankruptcy, domestic violence emotional and psychological child abuse as well as drug and alcohol abuse.

She believes the reason mental health stigma exists, is because we don't know how to talk about it. "It is a language barrier and a lack of understanding that fuels ignorance; thus talking about the Stigma is counter productive. "I want people to remember and understand what it is really like to suffer a mental illness or have mental health issues, not that there are people out there who don't believe it" she says.

She now dreams of a world where chickens can cross the road without having their motives questioned, where a mental health advocate has more followers than the Kardashians.

Contact

WEBSITE: www.bipolarbarbie.com

FASHION COMPANY: www.attitudeapparel.com.au

INSTAGRAM: @the_bipolar_barbie

TWITTER: @bipolarbarbieau

FACEBOOK: facebook.com/thebipolarbarbie

YOUTUBE: www.youtube.com/c/bipolarbarbie

SNAPCHAT: mycrazydays

ONLY FANS: https://onlyfans.com/thebipolarbarbie

TIKTOK: @thebipolarbarbie

EMAIL: bipolarbarbieaustralia@gmail.com

Other Books by the Author

The Bipolar Barbie Diaries
- Vol. 1   DROWNING
- Vol. 2   HELL
- Vol. 3   LIMBO
- Vol. 4   LAB RAT
- Vol. 5   CONFESSIONS
- Vol. 6   RECOVERY

www.ingramcontent.com/pod-product-compliance
Lightning Source LLC
Chambersburg PA
CBHW050258010526
44107CB00055B/2087